"*There is plenty of bad news these days, but the good news is that there is most definitely a food awakening taking place, and Veganish has arrived at just the right time to lend a hand. If you want your life to be a statement of compassion, if you care about the planet and the life it holds, if you want to live a long, vibrant and healthy life, there is probably no step you can take more powerful than eating a healthy, plant-strong diet.*"

— JOHN ROBBINS,
AUTHOR OF *DIET FOR A NEW AMERICA*, *THE FOOD REVOLUTION*, AND OTHER BESTSELLERS

Praise for *Veganish*

"*Vegan*ish offers gentle advice for vegans and those considering that diet."
— *Publishers Weekly*

"*Vegan*ish is more than just a cookbook. It's an open invitation to listen to your body's real needs and make healthy eating choices that go beyond labels. Mielle is magnificently authentic as she integrates both resourceful recipes and self-awareness."

— Tiziana Alipo Tamborra,
somatic experiencing practitioner and co-author of *Sweet Gratitude*

"Mielle's book, *Vegan*ish, is a well-rounded and informative narrative of deliciousness. This approachable take on omnivorous cuisine will appeal to any eater. A great book for anyone wishing to elevate their diet and create in the kitchen. The recipes are comprehensive and easy to use. I love this book!"

— Chandra Gilbert,
executive chef of the popular Los Angeles restaurant Gracias Madre

vegan*ish*

THE OMNIVORE'S GUIDE
TO PLANT-BASED COOKING

BY MIELLE CHÉNIER-COWAN ROSE

VIVA
EDITIONS

Published in the United States by Viva Editions, an imprint of Cleis Press, Inc., 2246 Sixth Street, Berkeley, California 94710.

Printed in the United States.
Cover design: Scott Idleman/Blink
Cover photograph: iStockphoto
Text design: Frank Wiedemann

First Edition.
10 9 8 7 6 5 4 3 2 1

Trade paper ISBN: 978-1-936740-84-0
E-book ISBN: 978-1-936740-97-0

Library of Congress Cataloging-in-Publication Data

Rose, Mielle Chénier-Cowan.
  Veganish : the omnivore's guide to plant-based cooking / by Mielle Chénier-Cowan Rose. -- First edition.
      pages cm
  Summary: "This utterly unique "vegan +" cookbook offers over 100 easy-to-make vegan recipes, many basic methods and cooking techniques, as well as advanced options. A trained chef, author Mielle Rose also offers pages of sage advice about food and nutrition, along with her personal story about transitioning from a 20 year long vegetarian diet to eating some animal-based foods"-- Provided by publisher.
  ISBN 978-1-936740-84-0 (paperback) -- ISBN 978-1-936740-97-0 (ebook)
  1. Vegan cooking. 2. Vegetarianism. 3. Cooking (Vegetable) I. Title.
  TX837.R824 2014
  641.5'636--dc23
                                    2014023123

Disclaimer
This book is not intended as a substitute for the medical advice of a licensed physician or dentist. The reader should consult a licensed professional in matters relating to his/her health and particularly with respect to any symptoms that may require diagnosis or medical attention. All suggestions regarding medical, dietary, political, and legal subject matter are based upon the information, belief, and personal opinions of Mielle Chénier-Cowan Rose only and should not be construed as directed advice. The ideas, suggestions, and procedures contained in this book are not intended as a substitute for expert assistance. Any application of the recommendations set forth in this book is at the reader's discretion and sole risk. Although the author and publisher have made every effort to ensure that the information in this book was correct at press time, the author and publisher do not assume and hereby disclaim any liability to any party for any loss, damage, or disruption caused by errors or omissions, whether such errors or omissions result from negligence, accident, or any other cause.

Dedicated to my family, and especially to my daughter Clara Rose. May your health continue to thrive, and may you always understand what there is to be grateful for.

I also dedicate this to you, dear reader, with blessings for you and your family's exceptional health and well-being.

Let's remember to give gratitude every day for the gifts that sustain us.

TABLE OF CONTENTS

Introduction

I was a devoted vegetarian for twenty years, and during the last twelve I was exclusively vegan. I spent those years learning and teaching about natural foods and began cooking professionally in 2000 as my practice of activism, to demonstrate the ease and pleasure of a plant-based diet. I earned my culinary certificate from Bauman College, an institute of holistic nutrition and healing culinary arts in the San Francisco Bay Area. I thank my career choice for my excellent health, because the natural restaurants and retreats I cooked for provided effortless access to fresh juices, wholesome meals, supplements, and cutting-edge health information while I was following such a restricted diet.

During those years, I would have protested anyone using the term *restricted* to describe my vegan diet. I've always enjoyed food enthusiastically and never lacked for inspiration from the plant world. Friends and colleagues often questioned whether I would partake if I could raise my own animals, but I could never give an easy answer. I relish animal-based foods as much as any gastronome, and was never fundamentally opposed to the natural course of life-taking-life-to-sustain-life, which indeed occurs in a plant-based diet as well. My complaint was, and still is, with the heartless practices of modern animal husbandry. I don't believe that humans have a right to treat sentient beings the way we treat most farm animals. We cannot possibly thrive by consuming the product of such intense suffering.

During the course of my vegetarian diet, the bigger question in the back of my mind was how I would handle a health threat that called for me to consume animal products—and eventually I found my answer. When a dentist prescribed surgery for my two-year-old daughter's severe tooth decay, with no promise of actual healing, I had to find a better solution. I discovered that tooth decay is linked to nutritional deficiency, and is somewhat common among vegan children. We began a healing regimen based on a book titled *Cure Tooth Decay*, which restricts grains, beans, nuts, and seeds and uses plenty of bone broths and marrow, raw dairy, and organ meats. My daughter's condition improved astonishingly quickly.

I am now a reluctant omnivore, humbly and gratefully using animal products to heal my family. I would prefer to hunt wild, free animals for our meat, but for the time being I have settled for hunting through information, seeking the most honorable farms and learning about which industry practices can—or can't—be avoided (see ABOUT ANIMAL-BASED FOODS). I am grateful for the farmers who do their best to give their animals a decent life and an honorable death.

I continue to grapple with my choice to include animal-based foods in our diet, yet I am not willing to risk my daughter's long-term health for the uncertainty. This choice has been bizarre yet empowering as I endeavor to heal my family and serve our meals with respect and love. I expected to raise my daughter with vegan principles, but now it seems I am charged to teach her about the dilemma of using animals for our nourishment, even as our diets will surely continue to change course. Learning how to cook with animal-based foods while writing a vegan cookbook has humbled me and opened my heart, and I strive to walk gracefully on the narrow path of such a paradox.

Indeed, a plant-based diet is cleansing and healing, both physically and spiritually, and some steadfast, long-term vegans do thrive. I believe it fosters compassion and peacefulness, and I have witnessed it heal life-threatening diseases. Nutritional needs change through different phases of life, though, and many people may need occasional animal-based foods to maintain optimum health in times of growth or recovery. If this is indeed true, we who rely on them must find ways to truly husband the animals that serve us. They deserve to be cared for with the greatest tenderness, respect, and gratitude we can muster. We must support and buy from the farmers and ranchers who are raising animals with this ethic. We must learn the traditional ways to use their entire bodies to honor the life that is taken. And we must become moderate in our consumption, for their sake as well as our own. This is key.

By now, most people understand that a healthy diet includes more vegetables and natural foods than the Standard American Diet (S.A.D.) provides. The inhumane yet ingenious model of the factory farm has made it possible for modern people to consume unnatural quantities of animal-based foods, and it's making us spiritually and physically sick. Nutritional recommendations change constantly, though, and the conflicting advice from multiple sources can be perplexing, especially when the latest discoveries are distorted into marketing hype for the food industry. Promoters of all sorts of diet trends—including the FDA—have led and misled generations of earnest eaters. We now have very convincing evidence for the benefits of vegetarian, vegan, and even raw plant-food diets, but another perspective holds to studies showing that elements of traditional diets that rely heavily on animal-based foods are critical to good health. One diet advocates meat but eschews grains and dairy, and yet another is mostly vegan while balancing ingredients according to energetic principles and seasonal changes. These diets and many others claim incredible health benefits and are promulgated with accounts of miraculous healing. As different as they all may seem, they do share common ground: an emphasis on plenty of vegetables and pure, natural foods.

What is pure and natural food? The answer can be somewhat subjective, but it implies food grown without chemicals and not adulterated beyond what's possible in an average home kitchen. Labels on packaged foods are not reliable guides for healthy choices, so we're left to our own devices to navigate the grocery aisles. My best advice is to eat a wide variety of naturally grown, unprocessed foods, and pay attention to how your body feels.

Buy ingredients that you recognize from nature and cook your meals from scratch as often as possible. Make an effort to avoid unnaturally altered, refined ingredients. Be moderate, balanced, and flexible. Trust your intuition and maintain a healthy curiosity about what you find.

If you're like most Americans, you probably know that your health could be improved by eating more vegetables. This book will help you learn to enjoy plant-based foods—whether you choose to eat this way all the time or just want to fill the rest of your plate with nutritious vegan foods. These recipes make up my basic vegan repertoire, and are capable of supporting a plant-based diet, but they're also easily adaptable for omnivores and lacto-ovo vegetarians to serve with meat or dairy products. Avoid imitation meats or cheeses, though, since these products are usually made of unhealthy ingredients and are often unsatisfying anyway (see ABOUT QUALITY INGREDIENTS). I offer a few recipes for satisfying, healthy alternatives like Cashew Cheese and Tempeh-Apple Sausage, but if you continue to eat animal-based foods, try to use them as more of a flavoring than as a main course. Be judicious, but go ahead and add a little grass-fed ground beef to my chili recipe, replace oils with organic butter, or serve my recipes alongside wild fish or pastured chicken, if need be. Follow your heart. The techniques are universal, as well as the information about ingredients to watch out for while you're focusing on improving your health. You may also be interested in my discussion about humane meat and dairy labels in the section ABOUT ANIMAL-BASED FOODS.

If you already follow a vegan diet, you're going to love my recipes, but you may not like my story. I'm another ex-vegan reluctantly encouraging you to pay attention if you feel compelled to include animal foods in your diet. It's not a simple choice, but we mustn't shy away from complicated, challenging conversations like these. We are on the brink of a third-wave vegan dialogue that calls for courageous honesty, faith, and open-mindedness. The early vegan movement was so desperately passionate to get the message out and wake the public out of its stupor to see what had become of animal husbandry that the nutritional aspect was glazed over or exaggerated for many years. We asserted that it was nearly impossible not to get enough protein and didn't provide enough education about critical supplementation to keep vegans thriving. Many who did thrive were "cheating" occasionally, contributing to a dangerous and misleading climate of secrecy and shame. Now we've seen a trend of ex-vegans angrily speaking up about their failing health, and their ensuing recovery by adding animal-based foods back into their diet. Next up is a frank discussion about the nutritional complications of the vegan diet, and how we might reconcile them with compassionate food choices. I've found a few accounts of devoted vegans successfully recovering their health with professional help and intense supplemental therapy, so it appears to be possible in some cases. I am excited to see what changes this more candid approach may bring to vegan outreach.

I offer the title *Vegan*ish very lightheartedly. It is ambiguous, like pregnant-*ish*, and I don't mean to dilute the integrity of a vegan person's earnest commitment. I'm using it here to acknowledge the benefits of plant-based foods, to encourage better treatment of farm animals, and to imply that any meal can include elements of a compassionate diet, contributing to the well-being of all concerned. *Vegan*ish gives a lot of room to explore how plant-based foods can work for everyone.

When lowering our reliance on animal-based foods, we may attempt to approximate them in new ways. We have to change our expectations when preparing plant-based recipes intended to remind us of familiar animal-based foods—not lower them, mind you, simply change them. It would be unreasonable to expect cashews to have the same taste or texture as dairy cream. Let these types of recipes be defined by their own qualities so that you can genuinely enjoy the results. They are delicious in their own right!

Finally, please do not simply use this like a recipe book. This is a *cook*-book! I hope it will actually spend more time on your nightstand than in your kitchen. While I do offer many of my favorite recipes, my real intention is to steer you toward reaching your own potential as a confident, intuitive, and skilled cook. Follow the recipes as closely or as many times as you need, but I invite you to trust yourself to modify them according to the ingredients in your kitchen or in season at your market. Use the Follow Your Heart recipes to learn methods to create flavorful dishes.

Food preparation is not an exact science. Every carrot is unique, both in size and flavor, and the types of salt, oil, or pan you use can make a difference in how a recipe performs. As with all recipes, merely allow mine to guide you in preparing fantastic meals that are personal to *you*.

I hope this book contributes something special to your relationship with food.

Mielle Chénier-Cowan Rose

About Plant-Based Nutrition

Let food be your medicine, and medicine be your food.

— HIPPOCRATES

Navigating all the nutritional advice available could drive a person to either obsessively examine their diet for all the correct up-to-date nutrients, or just throw up their hands and leave it to fate. In truth, you will probably be fine if you relax, follow your intuition, and pay attention to recommendations that resonate with you, and eat a wide variety of seasonal whole foods with joy and gratitude.

If you're watching your health, do your best to eliminate processed foods and focus on lots of leafy green vegetables and nutrient-dense whole foods. Digestive health is also very important so your system can absorb and use those nutrients. Fermentation improves the digestibility of many foods, such as soybeans (miso, tempeh), milk (yogurt) and vegetables (sauerkraut). Fermented foods also provide probiotics, which help digest and utilize the other foods we eat and strengthen our immune system to fight disease.

Fresh vegetable juice is an excellent way to consume a high dose of nutrients in one serving. Celery, cucumber, parsley and dark leafy greens are great choices. Limit higher-sugar vegetables like carrots and beets to accentuate flavor, rather than as a base. Ginger, apple, and lemon are great for flavor too. One of my favorite combinations is celery, grapefruit, and ginger.

Smoothies are a popular way to make a meal in a cup, but beware most commercial protein powders, which usually contain unnatural ingredients (see ABOUT QUALITY INGREDIENTS). Instead, use plenty of hemp seeds, nut butters, and spirulina to make high-protein smoothies. I always sneak some greens into my daughter's smoothies, too. A handful of dark leafy greens or sprouts, or a tablespoon of spirulina or therapeutic green powder blend such as Vitamineral Green makes a fruit smoothie exponentially more healthful.

Another cornerstone of a healthy diet is diversity. As much as possible, eat with the seasons, as nature intended. This ensures a wider variety of nutrients from multiple sources, increasing your chances of getting everything you need. Fruits and vegetables that are in season are more delicious, and are usually grown more naturally. Try to shop at farmers' markets or join a CSA (Community Supported Agriculture, a local farm box subscription model), and try new greens, roots, squash, and other vegetables when you see them at the market. This is more complicated during the winter months for folks who live in cold climates, so we can only do our best. Consider putting up some foods in late summer/early fall to get through the season, and just be reasonably mindful of the distance your food had to travel to get to your shopping cart. Kiwis flown from Australia in December might be something to pass up, but lettuce from a neighboring state is certainly something to be grateful for in the dead of winter.

When choosing supplements, try to buy those made from whole foods rather than those synthetically produced, or drink herbal infusions instead. Common nourishing herbs like nettles, oat straw, red clover, and comfrey are easily found at herb shops or online. Susun Weed offers easy instructions for brewing infusions on her website: www.nourishingherbalinfusions.com.

If you restrict your diet, it is especially important to give special attention to particular elements that could go missing. For instance, vitamin B12 has no reliable plant sources. Strict vegans must supplement this necessary vitamin, preferably taken sublingually and alone (as opposed to part of a multivitamin). Methylcobalamin is the most absorbable form of B12. It may also be important to supplement vitamin D on a vegan diet. If inadequate iron is a concern, vegetable sources include beets, pumpkin seeds, legumes, sea vegetables, and dark leafy greens. Eat these with a vitamin C-rich food to increase iron absorption.

Wholesome fats are very important to good health. They help absorb certain fat-soluble vitamins and maintain healthy nerves, hormone function, and brain development, among other purposes. Vegetable sources include avocados and unrefined coconut, olive, flax, hemp, and chia seeds, but it may be important to supplement DHA omega-3 fatty acids on a vegan diet. Quality vegan DHA supplements made from algae are available online, but some say that they must come from an animal source (such as fish oils) to be useful to the body.

I always include a stick or two of kombu when I cook rice or beans, because this mineral-rich sea vegetable provides lots of calcium. It also chelates heavy metals and radioactive minerals. Hijiki is another very high-calcium sea vegetable, one that is more delicate and should only be cooked briefly. All sea vegetables are rich in minerals and are great sources of iodine. (I recommend using natural sea salt, which may not provide sufficient iodine for some people.) Two other fantastic sources of calcium are unhulled brown sesame seeds and collard greens.

Try to eat dark leafy greens at almost every meal, which provide important minerals, vitamins, and micronutrients. I also eat a lot of cilantro and parsley. Parsley cleanses the blood, and cilantro chelates toxic heavy metals and radiation. Finely minced, these herbs can be tucked into sauces, dips, eggs, salads, soups, grains, and all types of dishes in large, therapeutic doses. (They are more palatable if you finely mince rather than chop.) Sprouts are a miracle food, which I discuss in more detail in the introduction to NUTS AND SEEDS. They have an incredible array of nutrients and a surprising amount of protein.

Quinoa is a reliable source of complete protein, which is crucial for vegans. Legumes, nuts, and seeds are other plant-based sources of protein. If whole grains make up a large part of your diet, they should be soaked, sprouted, and/or fermented before cooking, since their hulls contain an antinutrient that can inhibit mineral absorption (see introduction to GRAINS). This is particularly relevant to vegans and vegetarians who usually rely a great deal on grains for protein and calories.

If you are vegan but believe you might need some nutrition from animal-based foods, you may be encouraged to know that some of the most nutrient-dense, animal-based foods are the "by-products" of slaughter. (I am encouraged by this because I believe it's important to honor the sacrifice of life by using as much of the body as possible.) Organ meats, bone marrows, and bone broths are deeply nourishing and rebuilding, and make use of parts of the animals' bodies that are usually so disrespectfully wasted. Or, you can certainly experiment with how your nutritional needs could still be met by your vegan diet. The website www.veganhealth.org may be a good place to start. It is dedicated to helping people who are committed to a vegan diet find how they might make it work for their bodies. I've found that quality supplemental vitamins, minerals, and fats that are difficult to obtain from plants can be costly, and I believe that nutrients from whole foods are superior to extractions and synthetics, so for now I am resigned to using animal-based foods to heal my family.

If you are a committed omnivore but think you should eat less meat and dairy, you're probably right. The recipes in this book will help you make the transition away from the Standard American Diet (S.A.D.) that relies so heavily on them. Begin by using meat and other animal-based foods as a flavoring or side dish rather than as a main course, and allow nutrient-dense vegan foods most of the space on your plate. Be mindful of unnatural ingredients in commercial substitutes, though. I don't suggest you replace animal foods with fake meats or artificial cheese products. Most of these are made of chemically fragmented plant proteins and often contain genetically modified soy or corn ingredients. Burgers made from natural, whole plant foods such as fried tempeh, grilled portobello mushrooms, or beans and grains are delicious and satisfying. If you must have something more like meat perhaps just eat a grass-fed organic meat burger on occasion. It barely attends to the ethical dilemma, but in moderation, it may be a healthier choice for your body than a manufactured veggie burger. (Grass-fed and organic meats are both very important, as you'll see in the next couple of chapters.) Cashews and other nuts make very delicious "cheeses" and mylks, and tempeh is a nourishing whole food that can be crumbled and fried with seasonings in place of ground meats. Your efforts will be rewarded with increased vitality as you eat more plants and balance your system with wholesome foods.

Nutrition is very personal. Each body is different from the next, with its own individual requirements for functioning at its prime. Even a single body will have changing needs at different stages throughout its lifetime. It's wise to take note of nutritional recommendations and trends, but the best guide will probably be your own body's messages, telling you what it needs and how your diet and lifestyle are faring. Explore different nutritional models and allow yourself to shift between them as needed. Most diseases can be improved or even healed with changes in diet, so take charge of your health and find out what's necessary for you to thrive. Trust yourself to find the resources that you need, and remember the key factor of any healthy diet: a wide variety of fresh, unprocessed, naturally grown foods.

About Animal-Based Foods

• • • • • • • • • • •

To those who have hunger
Give bread.
And to those who have bread
Give the hunger for justice.

— LATIN AMERICAN MEAL BLESSING

Whether you are motivated to read a vegan cookbook by health, compassion, or curiosity, you don't need to be a sensitive animal lover to be moved by the gruesome violence inflicted on animals by typical farming operations. Even Julia Child, a staunch classical French chef, was moved to renounce veal when she was invited to a farm and saw the conditions firsthand. Most people would prefer to reduce animal suffering, including those of us who still choose to eat animal-based foods.

INTERPRETING MEAT AND DAIRY LABELS

Many concerned omnivores intend to support animal welfare with their purchases, but would be surprised to learn about standard practices on most "humane" farms. Reassuring but misleading labels such as *free-range*, *humane*, *cage-free*, *naturally raised*, and even *organic* allow for conditions that are rarely better than on the average industrial factory farm.

For example, most cage-free chickens live their entire lives inside grossly overcrowded barns. The label *free-range* is not much better; the range can be as paltry as a gravel courtyard accessed by a small door that most of the birds can't even reach through the sea of excrement and other chickens. Both labels allow painful beak cutting and forced molting through starvation. Organic labels require outdoor access, but the duration, quality, and amount is up to the farmers. There are no regulations for free-range cattle or pork. These, and organically raised cows, spend much of their lives in severely crowded feedlots, endure painful mutilations, and end their lives at the same high-volume slaughterhouses as conventional cows. These facilities are certainly not the pasture-grazing farms that compassionate consumers are hoping to support.

For the time being, **Pasture-Raised, Grass-Fed,** and **Grass-Finished** are more reliable labels for decent farm conditions. *Grass-finished* is important, because as the term *grass-fed* gains popularity, some farms are using it but finishing their cattle on GMO grains in factory farm feedlots. Certifications are helpful guides too. **Animal Welfare Approved** has the highest standards for humane practices, and **Certified Humane** is next best but does allow for beak cutting and indoor-only farms. **American Humane Certified** is fairly misleading, allowing for more painful procedures and small cages opposed by nearly every major animal welfare group in the US. The websites listed in SOURCES OF ADDITIONAL INFORMATION describe these labels and certifications. If you buy animal foods and want to make a difference with your purchasing power, do a little research so you can make your own choices about what is acceptable to you.

The term *natural* is one of the most misunderstood and misleading marketing claims on meat. It simply means that no artificial ingredients or preservatives are added, which is true for any fresh meat product. *Naturally raised* has a little more meaning, limiting hormones, antibiotics, and animal by-products in feed, but makes no mention of living conditions, so this often tricks well-meaning consumers into buying factory-farmed meat.

TRULY NATURAL ANIMAL-BASED FOODS

More humane farming conditions make for healthier animals, and healthier animal-based foods. Grass-fed and pasture-raised meat and eggs are leaner and contain more nutrients. The unnatural industrial diet of corn and grain—not to mention the unsanitary conditions of overcrowding—requires ongoing antibiotics to ward off disease. Conventional corn, soy, and alfalfa fed to most farm animals are virtually guaranteed to be genetically modified, which is proving harmful to animals and humans. In the previous chapter, I suggested that you eat an occasional burger rather than processed imitation meat foods, but the price of eating cheap, low-quality meat is just not worth it. More humanely and naturally raised animal foods do cost more, but we should eat them less often. In the long run, the health costs of cancers, diabetes, allergies, and other diseases will truly outweigh the grocery bill. The higher, fairer price of better farming conditions should compel us to eat fewer animal-based foods in the first place, which would be beneficial for most Americans' health.

SOURCING BETTER PRODUCTS

Grocery stores rarely sell truly pastured animal foods, but you can often find them at farmers' markets, from the farms themselves, or online. I still ask about their practices too, because even small farmers often cut beaks, horns, or tails, castrate, and apply third-degree burns for branding. These are painful procedures, all performed without anesthesia.

The websites www.eatwild.com and www.localharvest.org can help you locate sources for sustainably grown animal foods.

SAD NEWS FOR ETHICAL VEGETARIANS

Eggs and dairy products may be the cruelest of farming industries. What could be harmful about taking eggs, especially from a small, pasture-based farmer? To answer this, you must look back to where the chicks come from. Since egg-laying breeds are differentiated from meat chickens, male layer chicks are useless. Commercial hatcheries kill a quarter billion newborn males each year, and the standard practices are incredibly brutal. Farms of all sizes get their hens from these hatcheries, from the largest industrial operations to the smallest backyard farmers. Small, independent hatcheries do exist that sell the males to pasture farms for meat and do not painfully debeak the chicks, but they are rare. Some farmers still hatch their own chickens and raise the males for meat, but unfortunately a certain level of mistreatment is simply inherent to the production of animal-based foods, notwithstanding eventual slaughter.

Milk and cheese production also creates a surplus of male calves, which provide for the notoriously cruel veal industry. Even small farmers with only a few milking goats usually kill most newborn males, because they have no value. Female dairy animals don't have it any better, living to adolescence so we can exploit their procreative capacity. Within hours or days, CAFO (Concentrated Animal Feeding Operation, i.e. factory farm) farmers remove calves from their mothers, who bellow and search for their calves after they are separated, just as any human animal would in the same situation. Their lives are spent perpetually pregnant or milking until they are sent to slaughter when they cannot reproduce and give milk anymore. Industry slang crassly refer to the devices used to impregnate cows as rape racks, likely giving a good impression of the experience.

Vegetarians motivated by compassion for animals will probably want to consider all of this when choosing their diet.

> *The greatness of a nation and its moral progress can be judged by the way its animals are treated.*
> — MAHATMA GANDHI

About Organics

**The first step in making delicious food is to
use organically grown ingredients.
Really, they simply taste better.**

When you are accustomed to eating organic produce, you can taste the lack of vitality in conventional produce. Conversely, I've noticed that people who usually eat the Standard American Diet are often surprised to find that organics usually taste better. Some studies have revealed higher levels of vitamins and minerals in organic foods, which I believe contributes to their better flavor. I've found that if my recipes are not made with naturally grown ingredients, they may not taste like I intended.

Most people can agree that organics are important, but many are still put off by the higher cost. I share this concern myself, but I still prioritize organic food because of the vast hidden costs of industrial farming. Pesticides and herbicides harm farmworkers, contaminate groundwater, ruin soil, promote erosion, damage local ecosystems, and contribute to cancers and other health disorders. This does not merit my financial support. If you agree that quality food is worth prioritizing, consider looking for other places to trim your budget to accommodate the best foods for your family.

Farmers' markets are excellent places to shop for price. Local, seasonal produce often costs less than food that was grown hundreds or thousands of miles away, has a "greener" ecological footprint, and is even healthier, to boot. Organic labels aren't the ultimate marker for quality and sustainability: many small farmers grow their produce organically but choose not to pay the high prices for the bureaucratic process of organic certification. Farmers' markets are the best places to meet these independent farmers and ask questions about their growing practices. Their produce often costs less than the certified organic foods in the supermarkets. On this note, many brands of mainstream organic foods are owned by huge junk-food companies like Coca-Cola, Kellogg's and General Mills, which have financially supported measures that oppose GMO labeling and true well-being. Minimize packaged foods, even if they are organic. Whole foods made from scratch with naturally grown ingredients are healthiest, tastiest, and more affordable.

THE DIRTY DOZEN

The Environmental Working Group (EWG) publishes this list of fruits and vegetables found to have the highest pesticide residues even after washing or peeling. When making choices at the grocery store, these are the most important to buy organic or not at all:

Apples
Celery
Sweet bell peppers
Peaches
Strawberries
Nectarines
Grapes (imported)
Spinach/collards/kale/lettuce
Cucumbers
Blueberries (domestic)
Potatoes
Green beans

The EWG also publishes The Clean 15—a list of conventionally grown foods with the lowest pesticide residues—but here I urge us to consider more than our individual well-being. Poison has no place in the cycle of food production. We can take responsibility for our planet's future by choosing to support organic practices.

UNDERSTANDING ORGANIC LABELS

In the United States, the label **Certified Organic** indicates that a food was produced without antibiotics, hormones, pesticides, irradiation, or genetic engineering, and also dictates some animal handling and conservation methods. Labels marked as **100% Organic** mean that all of the ingredients are organic, while **Organic** means at least 95% organic ingredients were used, and **Made with Organic Ingredients** indicates that at least 70% ingredients are organic. The label **Non-GMO Project Verified** is an independent certification for products made according to best practices for GMO avoidance.

GENETIC MODIFICATION IS RISKY BUSINESS

Genetically modified organisms—GMOs, GM, or GE for genetically engineered—are almost ubiquitous in our food now, as yet unlabeled and largely unregulated in the United States. More than sixty countries recognize the risks of GMOs and have banned or restricted them, including Japan, Switzerland, France, Austria, Germany, Ireland, Mexico, and New Zealand. The US public is finally taking action, and as I write, states are making great progress in passing labeling laws and raising consumer awareness.

Animal tests and field studies show alarming reactions to GMOs, but politics and profits have kept them on the shelves. When GMOs emerged in the nineties, our government's own scientists saw the risks and recommended long-term safety testing, but corporate interests pressured the FDA to override and cover up their objections. Astoundingly, the government official who oversaw the lenient GMO policy was a former attorney for the Monsanto Company, by far the world's largest manufacturer of genetically modified crops. He returned to Monsanto as a vice president, and is now back at the FDA as a senior advisor of food safety. This is only one of the many glaring examples of the deep-seated conflicts of interest between the food industry and those who regulate it.

GMO safety testing is voluntary. The industry funds its own research, manipulates the scientific process, and suppresses unacceptable findings. Independent scientists are being censored and denied funding by their sponsors, under pressure from a complex system of corporate-political power. Some call this "tobacco science," likening it to the tobacco industry's manipulation of experiments showing that cigarettes were safe and beneficial, before the truth was exposed.

One example of the many dangers of GMOs is the story of Bt corn. The pesticide gene inserted into this corn kills pests by rupturing their intestinal walls, causing toxicity in their bodies from leakage. Bt corn is pervasive in the Standard American Diet, and gut-related disorders seem to have skyrocketed since it was introduced in the nineties. Many sausage makers import intestinal casings, because the intestines of Bt corn-fed US livestock are too weak. Parents report that GMO-free and gut-healing diets are improving conditions like ADD and ADHD, autism, allergies, and learning disabilities, the statistics for which seemed to rise in tandem with the introduction of this GM food. These concerns have yet to be confirmed by scientific tests, but the coincidence is hard to ignore: genetically modified Bt corn is probably degrading the intestinal walls of more than just the pests, not to even mention the detrimental effects of increased pesticides used on these crops.

Pollens from GMO crops contaminate organic and non-GMO varieties, and farmers are noticing negative behavioral changes in their animals fed GMO grains, as well as digestive and reproductive problems. This technology is uncontainable, unpredictable, and dangerous, and we have allowed money and power, armed with talented public relations, to lead it into our food stream and ecosystem. This is self-destructive human behavior.

The Institute for Responsible Technology is a comprehensive online resource for learning more about genetic modification (www.responsibletechnology.org). It also produces a non-GMO shopping guide in print or as an iPhone app. By refusing to buy GM foods, we can contribute to reaching the economic tipping point it will take to push GM ingredients out of our food supply.

The following are the most common genetically-altered crops and foods at the present time. I only buy these foods when I can find them organically grown:

Corn*

Soy*

Canola*

Sugar beets* (the source of most conventional sugar)

Cotton/cottonseed oil*

Alfalfa (conventional livestock feed)

Hawaiian papaya

Summer squash

Meat and dairy from animals given GM feeds or injected with rbGH/rbST

*By-products of these GMO crops are so prevalent in prepared foods that they are almost impossible to avoid unless labeled **Non-GMO Project Verified** or **USDA Certified Organic.**

Eat organic food. Or as your great-grandparents used to call it, food.

— UNKNOWN

About Quality Ingredients

· · · · · · · · · · ·

Good food depends almost entirely on good ingredients.

— ALICE WATERS

The best cooks are not afraid of salt, fat, or sweetness, but they also know that these ingredients are not created equal. Salts, fats, sweeteners, and other ingredients vary widely in quality, and therefore in taste. Choose ingredients that are worth using.

As with organics, I've tested some of my recipes using prepared foods with some of the unnatural ingredients listed below, and the results are always noticeably inferior. You must read ingredient labels if you want to ensure that you are buying quality food that tastes good. The vast majority of packaged, processed foods contain ingredients that have been altered to the point of distortion, and they will affect the flavor and purity of your meals.

Read labels and try to recognize the ingredients in the products you buy. Do they sound like food? Be vigilant, because many popular health foods also contain poor ingredients. They are owned by big agribusiness companies that are profiting from the natural foods movement while using cheap, inferior ingredients. If you live in an area where your options are limited, consider purchasing online or making your own.

INGREDIENTS TO AVOID

The following ingredients are sure signs of a low-quality product. Plenty of information is available online if you want to learn more about these unhealthy "foods."

Artificial flavors or colors are often derived from crude petroleum and are linked to ADHD, cancer, and other disorders. Avoid ingredients with numbers (such as Red #40) or the word *flavoring.*

Artificial sweeteners, such as aspartame, Nutrasweet, AminoSweet, and Equal, are considered excitotoxins, which are linked to obesity, cancer, and sterility. Some are produced with genetically modified *E.coli* bacteria.

Chemical preservatives can impact the nervous and immune systems, and some (such as BHA and BHT) are banned in many other countries for their links to cancers and behavioral or other disorders. They make foods seem fresh, even after they've actually perished. Avoid "foods" that do not decompose!

Corn syrup, especially high-fructose, may also now be called corn sugar. Studies link this product to obesity, diabetes, and gastrointestinal and cardiovascular issues. It is virtually guaranteed to be made from genetically modified corn.

Hydrogenated oils, including partially hydrogenated oils, are highly processed, likely genetically modified, and are widely recognized to cause a range of health problems. Many **vegan dairy substitutes** contain hydrogenated oils.

Monosodium glutamate (MSG) is a chemical food additive derived from the amino acid responsible for the elusive *umami* flavor, which naturally occurs in savory foods such as roasted meats, fermented miso and soy sauce, cooked mushrooms and tomatoes, and aged Parmesan cheese. Synthetically produced MSG is a potentially harmful neurotoxin that may overstimulate the nervous system. It is linked to obesity; some people report allergies, migraines, and even seizures when exposed to MSG. Many ingredients in **vegetarian meat and cheese substitutes** and **protein powders** contain synthetically produced MSG: soy protein, soy protein isolate, isolated soy protein, hydrolyzed vegetable proteins, autolyzed protein or yeast, sodium caseinate, modified food starch, and textured vegetable protein (TVP). A popular soy sauce substitute sold in health food stores may also contain this type of ingredient.

Meat substitutes are usually made of chemically derived plant proteins (see MSG, above). Seitan is pure wheat gluten, making it a more natural meat substitute that can even be made at home, but gluten is the protein in wheat that is most problematic for many people's digestion, so it will not be nutritious for everyone.

Natural Flavors is a misleading term that food producers can use to hide synthetically produced MSG (see above). It can include yeast extract, chicken flavor, and other flavors. Even if a package states "No MSG" on the label, it can still contain this type of ingredient. While some natural flavors may actually be real spices or seasonings, this designation usually indicates a synthetically produced chemical derivative of a previously natural element.

MISLEADING LABELS

In addition to the ingredients listed above, healthy shoppers must be aware of deceptive language on food labels. The USDA does not regulate many common terms that manufacturers may use to misrepresent unwholesome foods.

The term *natural* is meaningless, except on certain meat and poultry products. Other misleading terms include *pure* and *no artificial ingredients*; the latter gives the impression that a product is wholesome, yet the ingredients may still be altered beyond recognizable forms of their natural states. *Enriched* or *fortified* merely indicates that a manufacturer has removed nutrients from the original ingredients and replaced them artificially. Our bodies don't absorb this type of nutrition efficiently. The reassuring terms *free-range, humane, cage-free,* and even *organic* insinuate that animals have lived peaceful, natural lives on pastures, free of painful mutilations and unnatural living conditions. The reality is usually quite the opposite (see ABOUT ANIMAL-BASED FOODS).

About Salt

**Natural salt is vital to our well-being.
It helps regulate the water in our body and supports
the nervous system.**

Unrefined sea salt provides about eighty trace minerals, many of which are now missing from our foods due to depleted soils. In moderation, it is an essential element in a healthy diet. If you're concerned about sodium, you should remove packaged foods from your diet and start using quality salt at home. The flavor is more fulfilling, so you will need less, and you can gradually adjust your palate to appreciate less salt overall.

If you have a box of ordinary table salt in your pantry, move it under the sink and use it to clean your house. It is not a food. The taste is sharp and one-dimensional, and it's refined with bleach and chemicals to remove trace minerals. Anti-caking chemicals are added to keep the product from absorbing water ("When it rains, it pours"). This keeps the salt from doing its primary job in the body, which is to regulate cellular hydration. Unrefined salt is much better for your body and is better tasting, but it may clump because it's a natural product that absorbs water from the environment. Add a few grains of uncooked rice to a shaker of unrefined salt. These will absorb some excess moisture and make the salt easier to pour.

When you eat refined foods such as flour, sugar, and salt, you create a cycle of depletion and imbalance. Your body will crave more of the same empty foods, perhaps instinctively seeking the nutrients that have been removed. When we overconsume salt, our body sacrifices water from its cells to eliminate the excess sodium, leading to imbalance and illness.

Salt isn't just salty; it enhances flavor, even in sweets. Nurturing an intimate relationship with quality salt can help you become more intuitive in your cooking. Most chefs measure salt with their fingers, which I recommend. The physical contact with the crystals seems to tell me know how much I need. Add a little salt along the way as you cook to develop flavors from the get-go, and use salt to draw moisture out of vegetables as you sauté. Salt your blanching water "like the sea" to heighten flavors of the vegetables.

Pure, whole salt doesn't need to cost much more than the cheap stuff, and is well worth it. These salts come in a variety of textures and colors depending on the minerals present. Many natural chefs and home cooks swear by Himalayan crystal salt or Celtic sea salt. I love the texture and taste of Lima salt from France. Even if the label says sea salt, it may still be refined salt with chemical additives unless the package clearly states that it is unrefined. Find the ones that feel and taste good to you, but always read the ingredients label to make sure they are **unrefined** and **contain no additives.**

About Cooking Oils

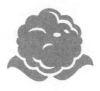

**I buy organic oils,
because pesticides accumulate in fat molecules.**

**I buy them in glass containers,
because fat degrades plastic,
which can cause toxic chemicals to leach into the oil.**

Fat lends important flavor and body to good food, but should be used wisely. Avoid bland, overly refined oils and instead choose nutritious fats like the oils listed below. Olive oil, coconut oil, seed and nut oils, and quality animal fats provide important fat-soluble vitamins, which support hormonal and immune health.

Choose an oil suitable for the cooking method you will be using. Consider flavor, but perhaps even more importantly, consider your cooking temperature. Heat degrades fat into carcinogenic compounds. The temperature at which this occurs is called an oil's smoke point. Refined oils have higher smoke points and can be used with higher heat, but unrefined oils have a fuller flavor and are more wholesome. Use these over low to moderate heat.

When you use refined oils, choose those that are naturally (mechanically) refined. Mass-marketed, generically labeled vegetable oils or cooking oils are refined using very high heat and toxic chemicals, and are undoubtedly made of genetically modified ingredients. Margarine and other industrial butter substitutes are not healthy choices, so if you are committed to a buttery taste, just use the real thing: delicious organic butter.

Store cooking oils away from heat, light, and air to prevent them from going rancid. Keep them tightly capped in a dark cupboard away from the stove or in the refrigerator.

I usually stock the following oils in my pantry:

Extra virgin olive oil: Naturally produced olive oil is very healthy. I use two types, a high-quality one and a mid-range one. High-quality olive oils have a strong fruity or nutty flavor. You can cook with these at lower temperatures, but heat will usually ruin their wonderful aroma. I save these more expensive olive oils for salads and finishing drizzles in soups, or over other dishes where the flavor stands out. Mid-range quality EVOO has a milder olive flavor. You can use this for low to medium-heat cooking, or substitute anywhere the higher quality would be used. Note that cheap "light" or "pure" olive oil has been denatured by refining.

Coconut oil can be used with any heat, and is a very healthful cooking oil. It is great for baking and useful as a substitute for shortening. Refined coconut oil is flavorless and more versatile, but I prefer unrefined for the sweet aroma and purity. See the GLOSSARY for more notes about its health benefits.

Light sesame or **peanut oils** are good for cooking at higher temperatures, with flavors that complement Asian dishes. When I don't have one of these on hand, I use coconut oil.

Safflower, sunflower, or canola oils have fairly neutral flavors and are interchangeable for cooking, baking, and salad dressings. Use unrefined for low-to-medium heat, and naturally (mechanically) refined for higher heat. I usually use coconut oil or one of these when the type of oil called for in a recipe is not specified. These oils are overconsumed in the Standard American Diet, and it bears repeating that canola is almost certainly contaminated with GMOs, whether organic or not.

Toasted sesame oil is not for cooking. This is a high-flavor finishing oil that I reserve for Asian dishes, especially Japanese ones.

Flax, hemp, and primrose oils are also not meant for cooking, but rather for using as a nutritional supplement at the table or in salad dressings. Store these in the refrigerator, because they go rancid easily.

Animal-based fats such as butter, ghee, lard, tallow, and duck fat are once again the subject of nutritional debate. For decades, both vegetarian sources and mainstream nutritional guidelines have asserted that saturated fats and cholesterol lead to disease, but rising evidence suggests that—in moderation—these are not only beneficial but crucial to good health. Ghee and tallow are very stable, and can withstand high-temperature cooking.

About Cooking Materials

The materials in pots, pans, utensils, bowls, strainers, and storage containers can break down and leach chemicals into your food. I've heard accounts of pet birds dropping dead when exposed to undetectable fumes from heated Teflon. Read on for my comments about common cooking materials, from the least to most reactive.

Glass is the safest, most stable material for food storage. Jars work well for this on a budget. Glass is also a good choice for cookware, as well as ceramic and enamel with lead-free glazes.

Wood cooking utensils are the least reactive choice. Stainless steel is the next best.

Cast-iron pots and pans are great, and they can even contribute iron to your food. They require a little extra care, but well-seasoned cast iron is as easy to use as nonstick pans and excellent for distributing and holding heat. Seasoning instructions are easily found online.

Stainless steel is strong and a good choice for pots or pans. All-Clad is very efficient and can be used with much lower heat to perform like a nonstick surface. Do not scour stainless steel; instead, cover burnt food with baking soda and a little water and simmer until the food loosens, scraping with a wooden utensil. Do not store highly acidic foods in stainless steel.

Copper conducts heat very well, but check that the protective metal coating is not scratched. Use the baking soda trick above instead of scouring. Don't cook with old copper pots, because manufacturers used to coat copper with nickel or tin, which leach easily.

Silicone is still considered safe, but no long-term studies have been conducted. My intuition tells me to avoid using it with heat. Some silicone products will show white streaks when twisted, which indicate cheap filler materials. These compromise the integrity of the silicone and have been reported to put an odor into foods, which can't be good.

Aluminum can seep into your food, particularly leafy greens and acidic vegetables. Dents and scratches on food surfaces increase the likelihood of contamination. Anodized aluminum is more durable and less likely to leach unless it is chipped, peeling, or scratched, but it is still a potentially harmful material. The safest aluminum cookware is coated in stainless steel anywhere food will contact it.

Nonstick coatings contain plastic polymers that give off toxic fumes when heated. A well-seasoned cast-iron pan is just as nonstick as these surfaces, and much better. You can also cook your food at lower temperatures with additional liquid to get the "nonstick" experience on other surfaces.

Plastic wrap, containers, utensils, and colanders deteriorate and leach carcinogenic and hormone-disrupting chemicals into your food, especially when heated. The more flexible the plastic, the more unstable the material. Use metal or wood instruments instead, and never use plastic with warm or hot foods. Do not store oily or fatty substances in plastic, because the oils further degenerate the material. Most canned foods have a plastic lining, but some have begun using BPA-free materials. Some vinegar and wine producers age or bottle their products in plastic, which is particularly dangerous with these acidic liquids. Look for those aged in wood and packaged in glass.

TECHNIQUES

Basic Cooking Tips

If you bake bread with indifference, you bake a bitter bread that feeds but half a man's hunger.

— KAHLIL GIBRAN

Enjoy yourself—no other technique is more important! Your attitude affects the food you prepare as much as your ingredients, and so cooking presents an opportunity to nourish your friends and family with your loving, positive energy. Make an effort to feel good in the kitchen and put aside any anger or frustration unless you can effectively transmute it into spiciness!

Trust your intuition. The more you can do this, the easier it will be to enjoy yourself. Eating is to cooking just as walking is to dancing, so relax. When something's in the oven, heed the voice that tells you to check on it. If you have an idea to add something different to your stew, notice where the idea originated. The voice of intuition will guide you and become stronger as you learn to perceive and trust it.

Read the entire recipe before you begin to cook. It's like looking at the map before beginning a trip. You will see what needs to be prepared ahead or how you can multitask along the way, making your journey through the recipe more efficient, easeful, and pleasant. You don't want to get stuck having to soak nuts overnight when you're trying to make dinner in an hour.

Mise en place is a French culinary phrase that literally means *putting in place*. It means measuring, washing, cutting, and otherwise preparing the ingredients for your recipe before you begin. This will also help you accomplish the previous technique, since you will need to read through the recipe in order to prepare your ingredients.

Maximize energy—your own, and that of your stove. When the oven is hot, roast an extra squash, a few bulbs of garlic, some tomatoes, or toast a tray of seeds or nuts. When you prepare beans or grains, double or even triple the quantities, so you can freeze leftovers. Try to make a few batches of sauces or salad dressings once a week. You will find it easier to prepare quick weeknight meals that are more complex and interesting with these building blocks on hand.

Essential Techniques

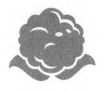

To **blanch,** or **parboil,** immerse vegetables in boiling water briefly, either to serve them al dente or to continue cooking with another method. Most vegetables appreciate this treatment before stir-frying, grilling, or adding to a stew to keep the flavors distinct and the vegetables firm. Blanch and then shock (see below) vegetables such as broccoli and cauliflower prior to serving with dips. When parboiling vegetables, I often salt the water heavily so that the vegetables take some on, making the final dish more complex. The water should taste as salty as the ocean.

To **shock** blanched vegetables, plunge them immediately into a bath of ice water. This stops the cooking process and keeps them bright and firm. I use this technique most often for broccoli to retain its color and crunch, but it's important anytime you want to keep your blanched vegetables from getting dull or overcooked.

To **deglaze** a pan after sautéing, add some wine, chopped tomatoes, lemon juice, or other acidic liquid to loosen the flavorful caramelized bits and juices from the bottom and incorporate them back into the dish. I usually do this before moving on to make a soup, sauce, or risotto. Use a liquid that will complement the final dish.

To **emulsify** a salad dressing so it stays creamy and blended, first combine all ingredients except oil in a blender or large bowl. Taste to make sure you have enough salt and that you like the flavor. Next, turn on the blender and add the oil *very slowly* in a stream while the blender is running (or begin to whisk vigorously in the bowl). Continue blending for thirty seconds or so after you've added all the oil. The best proportion of vinegar to oil is usually one part vinegar (or citrus juice) to three parts oil, but this needs to be adjusted according to the strength of the vinegar (see *Follow Your Heart Vinaigrette*).

Seek a **balance** of all the basic tastes in your menus (sweet, sour, salty, bitter, savory/umami, and pungent/spicy), and sometimes even within an individual dish or sauce. To correct and balance these in a dish or menu, you can use these guidelines to add something to the dish itself, or to inspire a harmonizing condiment:

Sweetness: sugar, honey, agave, fresh/dry fruits, stevia
- Balance with something sour, spicy, salty, creamy, or bitter.

Sourness: vinegar, citrus, tamarind, pickles, berries. Sour can reduce the salt needed in a dish.
- Balance with something sweet, salty, bitter, or creamy.

Saltiness: tamari, miso, sea veggies, celery
- Balance with something sour, sweet, or creamy. If you've over-salted a soup, you can dilute it with a little water, or boil a raw potato in it, peeled and quartered, to absorb some of the salt. Discard the potato pieces after about ten minutes.

Bitterness: dark leafy greens, lettuce, basil, cumin, coffee. Bitter often denotes healthful, alkaline foods/herbs.
- Balance with something sweet, sour, creamy, or salty.

Spiciness, or pungence: chilis , garlic, ginger, mustard, onion
- Balance with something sweet, sour or creamy.

Creaminess: coconut milk, oils, nuts, avocado, dairy.
- Balance with something sour or dilute with liquid.

Special Techniques

To separate **cauliflower** florets, cut the head into quarters through the stem. Lay each on its side on a cutting board and cut the stem off diagonally. The florets will come right apart.

To zest a **citrus** fruit, use a vegetable peeler if you don't have a Microplane or other type of zester. Zest is the super-flavorful, outer colored layer of skin on a citrus fruit. Shave off the zest and then use a sharp paring knife to trim away and discard any bitter white pith underneath.

To get the most *juice*, press and roll the whole fruit with firm pressure, then cut it in half and use a reamer or a fork to release the juices.

To *supreme* a citrus fruit means cutting the sections away from the membrane for a delicate salad or dessert. Begin by slicing off the top and bottom of the fruit. Stand the fruit upright and use a paring knife to cut away the peel and pith, following the curve of the fruit. Next, hold the fruit over a bowl and slice each wedge of citrus away from the membranes.

To replace **eggs** in a baking recipe, first determine their purpose. If they are in the original recipe to help bind the ingredients, you can replace each egg with any of the following: 1 tablespoon ground flax seeds briefly simmered with 3 tablespoons water (or blended until thickened) or ¼ cup applesauce, mashed banana, cooked squash, or mashed potatoes. If the purpose of the eggs is to give rise, use 1 teaspoon baking soda in the dry ingredients and 2 tablespoons vinegar in the wet, and bake immediately after mixing. If a recipe calls for more than 2 eggs, the results are unlikely to be very satisfying.

To choose an **eggplant** with fewer seeds, check the mark on the opposite end from the stem: a circle indicates a "male," and an oval or a flat line is a "female." "Female" eggplants tend to have more seeds, so you can avoid most of their bitterness and undesirable texture if you know how to pick out a male. Smaller eggplants tend to be less bitter as well.

To further reduce the bitterness of eggplants, you can toss raw slices with salt and let stand for 20 minutes, then blot dry before cooking. This is not necessary for Japanese eggplants and other small varieties.

When using **raw garlic or onion** in a recipe, I always refine the sharp flavor by marinating it briefly with salt and vinegar or lemon juice. It needs as much surface contact as possible, so a good garlic press or a Microplane to grate it is indispensable. Alternatively, you can crush the cloves, then finely mince them with a knife.

To roast **garlic**, slice the top off of a whole bulb and drizzle it with oil. Place in an ovenproof dish with ¼ cup water, and cover so it can steam. Roast at about 350° for about 40 minutes until cloves are soft enough to squeeze out the top. This is a delicious flavor boost to have handy, so roast a few bulbs at a time and store in the fridge or freeze.

To peel **ginger**, use a spoon to scrape off the peel. It's much easier than trying to do so with a vegetable peeler.

To soak **grains**, cover with lukewarm water and add per cup of grains a tablespoon of acidic liquid, such as lemon juice, vinegar, yogurt, or whey. This neutralizes some of the phytic acid, which can block absorption of minerals and protein. (Adding acidic liquid is especially important for strict vegans and those who rely heavily on grains in their diet.) Soak at room temperature for up to 24 hours, then drain, rinse, and cook as usual with slightly less water than normal. One cup of soaked brown rice usually cooks well with one and a half cups water, or one cup soaked quinoa with one cup water. Accelerated fermentation is an advanced method for brown rice that reduces up to 96% of the phytic acid after the fourth cycle. Simply reserve about a quarter cup of the soaking liquid each time you drain your rice, and add it to the soak water for the next batch. Refrigerate this "starter" liquid between batches.

Grain flours for baking can be soaked in the liquid called for in the recipe, replacing one tablespoon liquid per cup of flour with an acidic liquid. Soak for 12 to 24 hours, then proceed with the recipe. Do not try to drain the liquid from the flour.

To handle a **hot chile pepper** without burning your fingertips, use a fork to hold it while cutting or removing the seeds with a small, sharp paring knife. Taste each chile pepper for your recipe, because even if one is extremely spicy, the next may have no heat at all. Always wash your hands and utensils after working with hot chiles.

To finely chop **leafy herbs and greens** like parsley or kale, keep the bunch attached with the rubber band or tie. Wash under running water or swish in a water bath and shake off excess water. Holding the bunch together at the tips with one hand, begin to cut, moving your holding hand down the bunch as needed. If the herbs have a lot of stems, pluck off the leaves, roll them into a tight cigar, and slice into thin ribbons, called *chiffonade*.

To soak **legumes**, cover them with enough lukewarm water to double in size and add one tablespoon of salt per cup of beans to help with digestibility. Soak at room temperature for up to 24 hours, then drain, rinse, and cook with fresh water and aromatics.

To cut **matchsticks** of carrots or other round vegetables, slice long thin pieces (about ¼ inch thick), then lay flat to cut into thin sticks. This is also called *julienne*.

To soak **nuts and seeds,** cover them with enough lukewarm water to double in size and add one teaspoon of salt per cup to neutralize enzyme inhibitors. Allow to soak at room temperature for up to 24 hours, then drain and rinse. Store soaked nuts and seeds in the refrigerator for up to 3 days.

To toast nuts or seeds, place a single layer in a baking sheet or skillet and put in a warm oven (around 350°) or over medium heat on the stovetop. Stir occasionally until slightly browned and fragrant, usually between 5 and 15 minutes. Cooking times vary, so watch closely and heed your intuition.

To dice an **onion,** peel and slice off the top, leaving the root intact. Make four or five parallel lengthwise slices into it, but not all the way through the root, so that it holds together. Turn ninety degrees and cut the onion in half through the root, across the slices. Lay each half on a cutting board and cut crosswise across the slices; the small cubes will magically fall away.

To release **pomegranate** seeds, cut in half through the waist, rather than through the stem. Behold the sacred geometry. Hold one half in your hand over a bowl, seed side down, and spank it with a wooden spoon. They'll easily fall out into the bowl.

To roast a **red bell pepper,** place it whole over a flame or under the broiler, turning until almost completely black (up to 10 minutes each side). Remove it to a paper bag and seal the bag to keep in the steam. When cool enough to handle, pull off the blackened peels, stem, and seeds over a bowl to catch the sweet juices.

To peel a **tomato** for a very smooth sauce, slice an X in the end of the tomato opposite the stem and drop it in boiling water for 30 seconds. Shock in a bath of ice water, and then slide the peel off easily. This also works for peaches.

To open a **young coconut,** set it flat on the counter, take careful aim, and hit it with the sharp bottom edge of a large, heavy cleaver four to six times, around the top, to create an opening wide enough to scoop out the flesh. Lift off the top and carefully pour the water into a cup or bowl, then scoop out the flesh with the back of a metal spoon. Some people prefer to slice the white husk off the top first.

Menu Planning

**More often than not, I let region guide my menus.
Mama Nature knows how to turn us on, and she already
showed our ancestors how to do it with the plants
growing in each area.**

Menu planning is easier when you learn about international foods and the ingredients and seasonings used in different regions. There's no need to reinvent the wheel when composing a meal or a dish, because indigenous cultures already know how to expertly combine their native foods. Crossovers abound, of course, which allows for plenty of flexibility in combining regional foods and the creation of fusion cuisines. When experimenting with nontraditional combinations, keep it simple and engage just a few variables at a time. Maintain some underlying tone that keeps everything connected.

I am lucky to live in an area that grows a wide array of foods. I usually let the seasonal produce at my local farmers' market inspire me, thus allowing the Earth's natural guidance to nourish me. In this way, I eat a variety of wholesome foods over the course of the year, which is an important aspect of good health and creative menu planning.

A healthy plant-based meal typically features one or two protein-rich foods (presoaked legumes, grains, nuts, or seeds), with several vegetables, leafy greens, healthy fats, and a fermented food or other digestive aid. Take care not to overdo starchy foods: easy to do on a vegan diet. Strive for a variety of colors, which ensures an assortment of nutrients, and give attention to the textures on the plate, noting qualities such as crisp, crunchy, smooth, chunky, or tender.

Seek a balance of the five basic tastes in your menus, and sometimes even in an individual dish or sauce. These are salty, sour, sweet, savory, and bitter; Asian cultures add spiciness to this list. See ESSENTIAL TECHNIQUES for helpful tips about working with these flavors.

Finally, try to match the cooking method with the weather. Cool days call for longer, hotter cooking methods to warm us, such as oven roasting. In hot weather we need fresher, quicker methods such as steaming or even raw foods to cool us down.

Whatever you do to plan your menus, always prepare and present your food joyfully and confidently. Your food will reflect your intentions and your guests will appreciate your offering.

RECIPE PAIRING SUGGESTIONS

These lists will help you put together menus with a cohesive theme from the recipes in this book. Some of these recipes may not be completely traditional to the regions they are listed under, but they are close enough that they will complement each other when combined in a meal. Use the alphabetical INDEX OF RECIPES at the end of the book to find page numbers.

Southeast Asian (Thailand, Indonesia)

Coconut Jasmine Rice, Thai Green Curry Vegetable Stew, Carrot-Ginger Soup var. of *Simple Silky Zucchini Soup, Chilled Cucumber Mint Soup, Sesame Citrus Dressing, Thai Peanut or Almond Sauce, Sweet and Sour Glazed Vegetables, Spring Tonic Chee, Honey-Cayenne Pistachios* (use cashews or peanuts), *Tembleque Coconut Pudding, Indonesian Fruit Rujak, Dried-Fruit Compote* with ginger, *Market Fool* or *Chia Seed Tapioca* with tropical fruits, *Pineapple Rum Upside-Down Cake*

Indian

Coconut Masoor Dahl, Indian Curry Stew, Coconut Jasmine Rice, Chilled Cucumber Mint Soup, Carrot-Ginger Soup var. of Simple Silky Zucchini Soup, Honey-Cayenne Pistachios or cashews, Four-Flavor Mint Chutney, Fig Chutney var. of Peppery Fig Balsamic Dressing, Savory Chutney var. of Dried-Fruit Compote, Tembleque Coconut Pudding, Chocolate-Dipped Fruit var. of Chocolate Sauce (dried apricots are great), Rose-Scented Stuffed Dates, Rose Syrup over fresh fruit, Market Fool, Chia Seed Tapioca, Hippysauce Toast Spread

Japanese

Asian Braised Tempeh, Scattered Sushi Salad or Whole-Grain Sushi Rice, Creamy Dreamy Tahini Sauce, Sweet and Sour Glazed Vegetables, Simple Japanese Noodles, Japanese Kinpira Vegetables, Creamy Tahini-Coated Roasties, Rapini with Garlic and Lemon, Miso-Glazed Japanese Eggplant, Savory Roasted Shiitakes, Carrot-Ginger Soup var. of Simple Silky Zucchini Soup, Healing Hot and Sour Soup, Spring Tonic Chee, Lemon Tahini Dressing, Sesame Citrus Dressing, Tamari-Toasted Seeds, Gomasio Salt or 7-Flavor Seasoning var., Dried-Fruit Compote, Chia Seed Tapioca, Carrot-Tahini Butter

Latin

Follow Your Heart Enchiladas, Home-Cooked Black Beans, Polenta Four Ways, Summer's Glory Gazpacho, Smoky Black Bean or Butternut Squash Soup var. of Smoky Chili with Butternut Squash, Roasted Corn Chowder with Poblano Chiles, Chilled Cucumber Mint Soup, Secret Guacamole, Creamy Chipotle Dressing, Curtido Salad with Pepitas, Mission Pickles, Kipahulu Taco Sauce, Fresh Tomatillo Salsa Verde, Cashew Sour Cream and Cheese, Tembleque Coconut Pudding, Market Fool, Mayan Spice Cake var. of Heavenly Chocolate Cake, Dried-Fruit Compote, Chia Seed Tapioca, Chocolate Sauce

Mediterranean

Cannellini Beans with Tarragon, Quinoa Tabbouleh, Secret Hummus, Roasted Garlic Baba Ghanoush, Mhammara Red Bell Walnut Dip,

Olive-Pecan Tapenade with Pomegranate, Fabulous French Lentil Salad, Peppery Fig Balsamic Dressing and Marinade var., *Lemon Herb Vinaigrette, Balsamic Glazed Beets* and Orange var., *Spicy Roasted Cauliflower, Rapini with Garlic and Lemon, Roasted Root Medley, Spicy Roasted Cauliflower, Massaged Kale Salad, Marvelous Mushrooms with Wine and Herbs, Mushroom Risotto, Cashew Sour Cream and Cheeses, Simple Silky Zucchini Soup, Angry Cauliflower Potage, Summer's Glory Gazpacho, Chilled Cucumber Mint Soup, White Bean Soup with Kale, Balsamic Reduction, Nut Parm, Rose-Scented Stuffed Dates, Hazelnut Meyer Lemon Jewels, Market Fool,* Balsamic Glazed Figs var. of *Balsamic Glazed Beets, Heavenly Chocolate Cake, Cashew Dessert Cream, Dried-Fruit Compote, Chocolate Sauce, Chocolate Truffles,* Pasta Accompaniments (below)

Classic Americana

Follow Your Heart Wish Burgers, Homesteader's Honey Mustard, Simple Sauerkraut, Spicy BBQ Potato Salad, Creamy Coleslaw var. of *Curtido Salad, Tuna-Lover's Salad* and Tofu var., *Smoky Chili with Butternut Squash* or Soup var., *Skillet Cornbread, New Year's Black-Eyed Peas, Chicken-Fried Tofu,* Mushroom Gravy var. of *Cashew Hollandaise, Summer Benedict, Tempeh Bacon, Tempeh-Apple Sausage and Hash, Secret Guacamole, Honey Mustard Vinaigrette, Farmgirl Ranch Dressing, Cashew Sour Cream and Cheeses, Roasted Corn Chowder with Poblano Chiles, Simple Silky Zucchini Soup, Angry Cauliflower Potage, Wild Rice Pilaf with Cranberries and Pecans, Hazelnut Meyer Lemon Jewels, Market Fool, Heavenly* Chocolate Cake with Peanut Butter Frosting var. of *Chocolate Sauce, Dried-Fruit Compote, Chocolate Truffles, Chocolate Sauce,* Chocolate Dipped Fruit var. of *Chocolate Sauce,* Yellow Cake var. of *Pineapple Rum Upside-Down Cake, Lemon Cashew Cheesecake, Cashew Dessert Cream, Chia Seed Tapioca,* Pasta Accompaniments (below)

Holiday

Mushroom Risotto, Wild Rice Pilaf with Cranberries and Pecans, Rapini with Garlic and Lemon, Cannellini Beans with Tarragon, Roasted Root

Medley, Spicy Roasted Cauliflower, Balsamic Glazed Beets and Figs var., *Maple Balsamic Vinaigrette, Peppery Fig Balsamic Dressing, Marvelous Mushrooms with Wine and Herbs, Massaged Kale Salad, Mushroom Gravy, Mhammara Red Bell Walnut Dip, Olive-Pecan Tapenade with Pomegranate, Honey-Cayenne Pistachios, Cashew Sour Cream and Cheeses, Skillet Cornbread, Fabulous French Lentil Salad, Simple Silky Zucchini Soup, White Bean Soup with Kale, Angry Cauliflower Potage, Balsamic Reduction, Hazelnut Meyer Lemon Jewels, Rose-Scented Stuffed Dates, Lemon Cashew Cheesecake, Cashew Dessert Cream, Market Fool, Heavenly Chocolate Cake* or Yellow Cake var. of *Pineapple Rum Upside-Down Cake, Chocolate Truffles, Chocolate Sauce, Dried-Fruit Compote, Summer Benedict, Tempeh Bacon, Tempeh-Apple Sausage* and *Hash,* Pasta Accompaniments (below)

Pasta Accompaniments

Also try these recipes with polenta or over-cooked grains.

Nomato Sauce, Angry Sauce, Romesco Sauce var. of *Mhammara Dip, Parsley-Almond Pesto* or *Arugula-Walnut Pesto, Olive-Pecan Tapenade with Pomegranate, Raw Zucchini Pasta, Spicy Roasted Cauliflower, Marvelous Mushrooms with Wine and Herbs, Rapini with Garlic and Lemon, Cannellini Beans with Tarragon,* Creamy Pasta Sauce var. of *Cashew Hollandaise* with or without *Tempeh-Apple Sausage* or *Bacon, Nut Parm, Creamy Dreamy Tahini Sauce, Thai Peanut* or *Almond Sauce, Simple Japanese Noodles, Miso-Glazed Eggplant,* any salad dressing with less oil and steamed veggies

RECIPES

Salad Dressings

Your family will love eating their greens if the salad dressing is delicious. My five-year-old eats more salad than most adults with these dressing recipes!

Making your own salad dressing is so easy, and one of the best ways to care for your health and your food budget. Commercial salad dressings are filled with unwholesome ingredients and cost much more than they're worth (see ABOUT QUALITY INGREDIENTS). You can easily multiply these recipes to keep plenty on hand throughout the week when you need a quick, easy meal.

I use a blender to emulsify these dressings, but you can also do it with a fork or small whisk in a bowl if you add the oil slowly enough.

FOLLOW YOUR HEART VINAIGRETTE

Yields 1 cup

Read up about emulsification in ESSENTIAL TECHNIQUES and take note of the proportions. This formula sets you free to make your own dressing anytime.

Combine first in blender to dissolve salt:

¼ cup vinegar or citrus juice

1 tsp salt

Turn on blender and VERY SLOWLY add:

¾ cup oil (1 cup if using balsamic vinegar)

Continue blending up to 30 seconds to emulsify.

Notes

- Adjust this formula for the acidity of vinegar, using more oil with stronger vinegars. 4:1 balsamic vinegar, 2:1 rice wine vinegar, 6:1 sherry vinegar.
- You can mix oils and vinegars too. For example, a small amount of a strong nut oil stands out plenty with a mild olive oil, and a little balsamic is nice to temper stronger vinegars.
- To get a really good, lasting emulsification, add pressed garlic, mustard, tomato paste, cream, or egg yolks before the oil.
- If making a small batch, just add the ingredients in a bowl, drizzling the oil drop by drop while whisking vigorously to create an emulsion.
- Once a salad is tossed, taste again and add a little salt or vinegar if necessary for the perfect balance to your taste.

Vinegars

- Apple cider: all-purpose, slightly sweet flavor.
- Balsamic: sweet; different qualities vary widely from rich, thick aged varieties to acidic or too-sweet cheaper types.
- Champagne: delicate, complements tender greens like butter lettuce.

- Red wine: can be strong, good with olive and nut oils.
- Rice wine: mild, sweet, great with Japanese flavors. I prefer "unseasoned," which does not have added sugar.
- Sherry: very strong, great with nut oils and robust, bitter greens.
- White wine: somewhat delicate, best with neutral oils.

Oils

- Extra virgin olive: strong and fruity. Estate-bottled is pricier but worth it for salads.
- Sesame: light sesame is mild, dark is roasted and nutty, great for Asian flavors.
- Sunflower or safflower: mild and neutral
- Nuts (walnut, hazelnut, etc.): should smell fresh and nutty, not rancid. These are strong, and mix well with strong vinegars.

Variations

- Add savories such as freshly ground pepper, garlic, shallots/onions, ginger, fresh herbs, mustard, olives, capers, fresh or roasted tomatoes, or chile peppers.
- Add sweeteners such as honey, maple syrup, fresh or dried fruit, sugar, juice concentrates, or agave syrup.
- Replace some or all of the salt with miso or tamari (best with sesame or peanut oils and Asian flavors).
- Replace some or all of the oil with avocado, tahini, soaked nuts or seeds, or nut/seed butters.
- See MENU PLANNING for notes about combining ingredients to create a cohesive flavor.
- Vinaigrettes can also be marinades, especially if you add salt, wine, garlic, or extra acid element.

Omnivorous variations

- Soft cheeses, yogurt, mayonnaise, crème fraiche, cream, raw or boiled eggs, or buttermilk can replace some or all of the oil.
- Anchovies can be another interesting salty element.

LEMON HERB VINAIGRETTE

Yields 1 cup

This dressing is excellent on a classic Greek salad with thinly sliced red onion, chunks of cucumber and tomato, olives or capers, parsley, and the herbed feta variation of *Cashew Sour Cream and Cheeses* (NUTS AND SEEDS).

Combine in a blender:

1 tsp salt

1 clove garlic, finely grated

¼ cup lemon

Allow to marinate 5–10 minutes, then add:

1 tsp *Homesteader's Honey Mustard* (DIPS AND SPREADS)

several twists black pepper

up to ¼ cup fresh herbs: oregano, thyme, marjoram, parsley

1 tsp honey, agave syrup, or maple syrup (optional)

Turn on blender and SLOWLY add:

¾ cup extra virgin olive oil

Continue blending up to 30 seconds to emulsify.

Omnivorous variations

- Reduce oil to ¼ cup to use as a marinade for organic, pastured meats.
- Organic feta is a great complement to this salad dressing.

PEPPERY FIG BALSAMIC DRESSING

Yields 1½ cups

I created this recipe for the West Coast raw foods restaurant phenomenon Café Gratitude. A version of it continues to be a favorite there.

Soak for about 20 minutes:

6 dried figs, stems removed

just enough water to submerge

When soft, drain (reserve soaking water) and place in blender with:

3 Tbsp soaking water

¼ cup balsamic vinegar

½ jalapeño pepper, seeded

1 tsp salt

¼ tsp black pepper, ground

Turn on blender and SLOWLY add:

¾ cup extra virgin olive oil

Continue blending up to 30 seconds to emulsify.

Fig Balsamic Marinade variation

- Reduce oil to 2 Tbsp and add up to ¼ cup water to use as a marinade for tofu or vegetables.

Fig Chutney variation

- Omit oil to serve as a chutney or dipping sauce. Add water or lime juice as needed to achieve a good consistency.

Omnivorous variations

- Organic feta cheese is a nice complement to this dressing.
- Try whipping the chutney variation with organic cream cheese and chopped walnuts for a delicious cracker spread.
- The marinade and chutney variations above are great accompaniments to organic, pastured meats.

FARMGIRL RANCH DRESSING

Yields about 2 cups

Soaked cashews have a short shelf life, but this dressing is so good that eating it up in a day or two should be no problem. It is delicious as a vegetable dip too. I love using the herbs suggested, but you can get creative with whichever are growing in your garden or are currently at your market.

Cover with water and soak for at least 1 hour, up to 24:
⅓ cup raw cashews
2 Tbsp raw sunflower seeds
½ tsp salt

Drain, rinse, and set aside.

Combine in a blender:
¼ cup lemon juice or apple cider vinegar
1 tsp salt
1 small clove garlic, finely grated

Allow to marinate 5–10 minutes, then add:
soaked cashews and sunflower seeds, above
1 Tbsp tamari
2 Tbsp nutritional yeast
pinch cayenne
2 Tbsp water, more if needed

Turn on blender and SLOWLY add:
1 cup oil

Continue blending up to 30 seconds to emulsify, adding more water if needed for consistency. Stir in:
½ cup parsley, minced
2–4 Tbsp fresh dill, minced
2 Tbsp chives, minced
other fresh herbs as desired: cilantro, marjoram, basil, etc.

Nut-free variation

- Omit cashews and sunny seeds. Reduce oil to ¼ cup and add 1 cup mashed avocado.

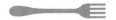

HONEY MUSTARD VINAIGRETTE

Yields 1 cup

This lighter version of a classic diner salad dressing is perfect on light greens with shredded carrots, raw walnuts, and apple cubes.

Combine in a blender:

¼ cup apple cider vinegar

1 tsp salt

1 tsp *Homesteader's Honey Mustard* (Dips and Spreads)

¼ cup honey

½ tsp poppy seeds (optional)

Turn on blender and SLOWLY add:

½ cup oil

Continue blending up to 30 seconds to emulsify.

Note

- Many vegans do not eat honey due to the inherent exploitation of bees. Replace it with 2 Tbsp maple or agave syrup if you prefer.

Omnivorous variation

- Substitute organic yogurt, mayonnaise, or sour cream for some or all of the oil. Adjust salt and vinegar as desired.

MAPLE BALSAMIC VINAIGRETTE

Yields 1 cup

I love this dressing anytime, and it really shines on spicy greens like arugula, or in a *Massaged Kale Salad*.

Combine in a blender:

¼ cup balsamic vinegar

2 Tbsp apple cider vinegar

2 tsp salt

2–3 Tbsp maple syrup

pinch freshly ground pepper

2 Tbsp *Homesteader's Honey Mustard* (DIPS AND SPREADS) (optional)

Turn on blender and SLOWLY add:

½ cup extra virgin olive oil

Continue blending up to 30 seconds to emulsify.

Maple Balsamic Marinade variation

- Reduce oil to 2 tablespoons to use as a marinade, braising liquid, or baste for finishing tofu, tempeh, mushrooms, and other vegetables.

Omnivorous variation

- The marinade variation above is also great for organic, pastured meats.

LEMON TAHINI DRESSING

Yields 1½ cups

This dressing stands up well to a *Massaged Kale Salad*, and you can also use it as a sauce for grains or vegetables if you prefer it instead of *Creamy Dreamy Tahini Sauce* (Sauces).

Combine in a blender:

juice of 4 lemons or limes (or ½ cup rice vinegar)

1½ tsp salt

Allow to marinate 5–10 minutes, then add:

½ cup tahini

½ cup water

Turn on blender and SLOWLY add:

¼ cup oil

Continue blending up to 30 seconds to emulsify.

Optional additions

- 2–4 Tbsp minced fresh herbs such as parsley, cilantro, chives, or basil
- 2–3 tsp honey, maple, or agave syrup
- 1 tsp grated fresh ginger, garlic, or both
- 2 Tbsp toasted sesame oil
- 2 tsp *Homesteader's Honey Mustard* (Dips and Spreads)
- juice of 1 orange
- pinch cayenne

Omnivorous variation

- You may substitute organic yogurt or buttermilk for the water.

SESAME CITRUS DRESSING

Yields 1⅓ cups

This is one of my favorite dressings, ever. I owe the inspiration to my first professional cooking job at Calistoga Natural Cafe. With less oil, it's a delicious marinade for blanched vegetables, tofu, or meat.

Combine in a blender:

¼ cup rice vinegar

grated zest of 1 lime and 1 orange

juice of 1 lemon, 1 lime, and 1 orange

1½ tsp salt

1 tsp grated fresh ginger

2 Tbsp honey

2 tsp tamari or shoyu

4 tsp toasted (dark) sesame oil

Turn on blender and SLOWLY add:

½ cup light sesame oil, or any light oil

Continue blending up to 30 seconds to emulsify.

Asian Marinade variation

- Reduce oil to 2 tablespoons to use as a marinade, braising liquid, or baste for finishing tofu, tempeh, mushrooms, and other vegetables.

Omnivorous variation

- The marinade variation above is also great for organic, pastured meats.

CREAMY CHIPOTLE DRESSING

Yields about 1 cup

This dressing makes an awesome potato salad (see *Spicy BBQ Potato Salad* in VEGETABLES), taco sauce, raw vegetable dip, or sandwich spread. The spiciness of the chile peppers will vary greatly, so start with less and taste before adding more. The heat will mellow as it stands.

Combine in a blender:

1 small clove garlic, finely grated

1 Tbsp apple cider vinegar

1 Tbsp balsamic vinegar, or the juice and zest of ½ orange

juice of ½ lemon or lime

¾ tsp salt

Allow to marinate 5–10 minutes, then add:

1–3 Tbsp chipotle paste, or 1–3 tsp chipotle powder

3 Tbsp tahini

2–4 Tbsp water, depending on consistency of tahini

2 tsp honey (optional)

Turn on blender and SLOWLY add:

½ cup oil

Continue blending up to 30 seconds to emulsify.

Omnivorous variations

- This recipe is also a delicious dip for organic, pastured chicken kebabs or homemade chicken nuggets.
- You can substitute organic yogurt or sour cream for some or all of the oil.

Sauces

I've found that sauce seems to be most people's favorite food! My vegan meals often rely on a fantastic sauce over simple beans, grains, and roasted or steamed vegetables. I've barely done anything, and yet people are easily pleased by the tasty smothering.

These other recipes can also be served as sauces or toppings, especially for pasta, polenta, or grains:

SALAD DRESSINGS: any, using less oil

DIPS: Romesco Sauce variation of *Mhammara*, *Olive-Pecan Tapenade with Pomegranate*

NUTS AND SEEDS: *Cashew Sour Cream and Cheeses*

VEGETABLES: sauce from *Raw Zucchini Pasta*, *Marvelous Mushrooms with Wine and Herbs*, *Rapini with Garlic and Lemon*

ROASTIES: *Spicy Roasted Cauliflower*, *Miso-Glazed Eggplant*

LEGUMES: *Cannellini Beans with Tarragon*

GRAINS: sauce from *Simple Japanese Noodles*

DESSERTS: *Balsamic Reduction*, Savory Chutney variation of *Dried-Fruit Compote*

BREAKFASTS: *Cashew Hollandaise*, and Mushroom Gravy and Creamy Pasta Sauce variations

KIPAHULU TACO SAUCE

Yields 2 cups

My sisters Jade and Patricia made sauces like this at their makeshift tamale stand in the Maui jungle. You'll put it on everything if you're a hot sauce junky like me.

Combine in a pan over medium-low heat:

1 onion, chopped

1 tsp salt

2 Tbsp oil

Cook about 10 minutes, until onions begin to color. Add:

2 cups tomatoes, roughly chopped

3 cloves garlic, minced

3 chipotle chiles (or any hot peppers), chopped

Cover and cook over medium heat for 10–15 minutes, stirring occasionally. Allow to cool, then place in a blender with:

juice of 2 limes (or ¼ cup apple cider vinegar)

Purée and adjust salt, lime, and chiles to taste. (Add water if necessary.) The heat will mellow as it stands.

Carrot Chipotle Sauce variation

- Substitute steamed carrots for the tomatoes.

FRESH TOMATILLO SALSA VERDE

Yields 2 cups

Chile peppers can be unpredictable, so adjust the quantity or remove the seeds, depending on how spicy they are. See SPECIAL TECHNIQUES for hints on handling them.

Blacken over a flame or under a broiler:

> 2 jalapeño chiles

Trim off stems and place in a blender with:

> ¼ yellow onion
> 2 cups tomatillos, husked
> 1–2 cloves garlic
> ½ bunch cilantro, chopped
> juice of 2 limes
> 1 tsp cumin powder
> 1 tsp salt

Purée and adjust salt and lime to taste.

Roasted variation

- Quarter the raw tomatillos and jalapeños. Toss with a little olive oil and salt and roast in a 425° oven for 25 minutes. Blend with remaining ingredients.

CREAMY DREAMY TAHINI SAUCE

Yields ½ cup

Tahini is a rich, creamy purée of calcium-rich sesame seeds. Serve this staple sauce over grains and cooked vegetables, as a dip for crudités, an oil-free dressing, or as the creamy element for vegan tacos. Add the water a little at a time, because it can become too wet very suddenly.

Use a fork or small whisk to combine in a bowl:

¼ cup tahini

1–2 Tbsp tamari, or ¼–½ tsp salt

2–3 Tbsp vinegar (rice or apple cider), or lemon or lime juice

Mix well, adding a tablespoon of water at a time to achieve a creamy consistency. Balance flavors to your taste (salty, sour, sweet, etc.).

Optional additions

- 1 clove garlic, grated*
- 1 Tbsp toasted sesame oil*
- Minced scallions, chives, or fresh herbs such as parsley or cilantro*
- 1 tsp grated fresh ginger
- juice of ½ orange
- 1–2 tsp honey or agave syrup
- Chile peppers or cayenne, to taste

*I almost always include these if I have them on hand.

Omnivorous variation

- You can add 1 cup organic yogurt to make a thin, creamy Middle Eastern sauce for falafel, roasted meats, or a chopped vegetable salad with chickpeas.

ANGRY SAUCE

Yields 4 cups

I borrowed this name from the spicy Italian sauce called Arrabbiata, meaning angry. More a ragout than a sauce, this recipe can be served with pasta or polenta, or as a bruschetta topping.

Preheat oven to 400°. Combine in a casserole dish:

2 lb Roma tomatoes, quartered or smaller

2 red bell peppers, sliced (optional)

1 red onion, thinly sliced

5 large cloves garlic, chopped

3 Tbsp capers, rinsed, or kalamata olives

¼ cup olive oil

1 tsp salt

freshly ground pepper

1–2 sprigs fresh rosemary, chopped

½–1 tsp crushed red pepper, to taste

Roast about 40 minutes, until saucy, stirring occasionally. Before serving, toss with:

¼ cup chopped fresh herbs (parsley, oregano, thyme, marjoram, rosemary, basil, etc.)

extra drizzle of a quality olive oil

splash of balsamic or lemon (optional)

Serve as is or purée for a smooth consistency.

Variations

- For a very smooth sauce, peel the tomatoes before cooking (see SPECIAL TECHNIQUES).
- Add *Tempeh-Apple Sausage* (BREAKFASTS).

Omnivorous variation

- If you want animal protein with this vegan sauce, add a little bit of cooked and crumbled organic, pasture-raised sausage.

ARUGULA-WALNUT PESTO

Yields 1½ cups

Pestos are versatile and can be served in many ways other than pasta. Try this as a soup garnish, over grilled or roasted vegetables, in a gratin or lasagna, as a sandwich spread, or add extra oil to make a dip for bread or lightly blanched vegetables.

Combine and allow to marinate for 5–10 minutes:

1 clove garlic, finely grated

½ tsp salt

juice of 1 lemon

Transfer to a food processor with:

½ cup walnuts, toasted (see SPECIAL TECHNIQUES)

1 bunch arugula leaves, chopped (about 2 cups)

Turn on processor, and slowly drizzle:

½ cup olive oil

Process to achieve a creamy consistency. Adjust lemon and salt to taste.

Variations

- Add up to ¼ cup nutritional yeast.
- Replace walnuts with pumpkin seeds.
- Make this recipe into a pistou (see GLOSSARY) by omitting the nuts and reducing the olive oil by half.

Omnivorous variations

- You can add ½ cup organic Parmesan cheese.
- This vegan pesto is great with fish or chicken too.

PARSLEY-ALMOND PESTO

Yields about 2 cups

Parsley is a very nutritious herb, high in vitamin C and cleansing for your blood. It grows easily in a backyard garden, and this recipe helps you use plenty. This makes a great dressing for potato or pasta salad.

Combine and allow to marinate for 5–10 minutes:

1 clove garlic, finely grated

½ tsp salt

zest and juice of 1 lemon

Transfer to a food processor with:

½ cup almonds, toasted (see SPECIAL TECHNIQUES), or almond butter

1 bunch parsley leaves (about 1 cup packed)

½ bunch basil leaves (about ¼ cup packed)

Turn on food processor and slowly drizzle:

½ cup olive oil (may add up to ½ cup more, to taste)

Process to achieve creamy consistency. Adjust lemon and salt to taste.

Variations

- Add up to ¼ cup nutritional yeast.
- Replace almonds with macadamias or pine nuts.
- Make this recipe into a pistou (see GLOSSARY) by omitting the nuts and reducing the olive oil by half.

Omnivorous variations

- You can add ½ cup Parmesan cheese if desired.
- This vegan pesto is great with fish or chicken too.

NOMATO SAUCE
··

Yields 5 cups

Use this as an alternative red sauce for pasta or pizza if you avoid night-shades, need extra iron from the beets, or just want something different. You can also serve it as a dip for bread.

Cook until soft (steam, boil, or roast in oven):
  4–6 large beets (about 8 cups chopped)

Set aside. Meanwhile, combine in a medium pot:
  1 tsp olive oil
  2 stalks celery, chopped
  1 yellow onion, diced
  ½ tsp salt

Cook over medium-low heat about 10 minutes, until onions begin to color. Add:
  3 large cloves garlic, minced
  ⅛ tsp crushed red pepper
  1 Tbsp dried Italian seasoning, rubbed between palms
  1 tsp fennel seeds, ground

Cook about 3 more minutes, until garlic is fragrant. Add:
  ¾ cup red wine

Deglaze pan (see ESSENTIAL TECHNIQUES) and simmer until pan is nearly dry again, then add:
  cooked beets, above
  ½ tsp salt
  ½ tsp black pepper
  6 Tbsp olive oil
  ¼ cup chopped fresh herbs (oregano, rosemary, parsley, thyme, marjoram, etc.)

Purée in food processor or blender, adding a little water or broth if necessary to achieve desired consistency. Adjust salt to taste.

Variation

- Add *Tempeh-Apple Sausage* (BREAKFASTS).

Omnivorous variation

- If you want animal protein with this vegan sauce, add a little bit of cooked and crumbled organic, pasture-raised sausage.

THAI PEANUT OR ALMOND SAUCE

Yields ½ cup

This popular sauce is delicious over vegetables and grains. It also makes a great dipping sauce for spring rolls, vegetable kebabs, fried sweet potatoes or tofu, celery sticks, or rice noodles. Notice that it's simply a variation of the *Creamy Dreamy Tahini Sauce.*

Combine in a bowl or blender:

2 Tbsp lime juice, or 1 Tbsp tamarind paste

1 tsp salt

1 Tbsp shoyu or tamari

¼ cup peanut or almond butter

½ tsp grated fresh ginger

1 tsp honey or agave syrup

1 Thai chile pepper or ⅛ tsp cayenne, to taste

1 tsp toasted sesame oil (optional)

Blend, adding a tablespoon of water at a time to achieve a creamy consistency. Add:

chopped mint or cilantro (optional)

Balance flavors to your taste (salty, sour, spicy, and sweet).

Omnivorous variation

- This vegan sauce is also great with organic, pastured chicken kebabs, or as a dressing for a chicken salad with mint and chopped veggies.

FOUR-FLAVOR MINT CHUTNEY

Yields about 1½ cups

I love Indian chutneys and sauces. I always combine them to achieve a flavor similar to this delicious dipping sauce: spicy, sweet, sour, and minty.

Soak for about 10 minutes:

½ cup raisins, or dried apricots

water to cover

When soft, drain (reserve soaking water) and place in a blender with:

1 bunch cilantro, chopped (about 2 cups loosely packed)

½ bunch mint leaves (about 1 cup loosely packed)

1 jalapeño or serrano chile, seeded

juice of 2 limes, about ¼ cup

½ tsp each cumin and coriander seeds, toasted

1½ tsp salt

¼ cup diced red onion or shallot (optional)

Blend until smooth, using the water from soaking the raisins as necessary to achieve desired consistency.

Variations

- Add 1 cup oil (see *Emulsify* in ESSENTIAL TECHNIQUES) to use as a dressing for hearty greens.
- Add only 2 Tbsp oil to use as a marinade for tofu or vegetables.

Omnivorous variation

- This vegan chutney and the variations above are great accompaniments to organic, pastured meats.

Dips and Spreads

'Tis an ill cook that cannot lick his own fingers.

— WILLIAM SHAKESPEARE

Serve these recipes as appetizers with crackers, bread, or crudités (raw or briefly blanched vegetables), or as spreads for sandwiches or raw wraps.

These recipes can also be served as dips or spreads:

SALAD DRESSINGS: *Peppery Fig Balsamic Dressing, Farmgirl Ranch Dressing, Creamy Chipotle Dressing, Lemon Tahini Dressing*

SAUCES: *Kipahulu Taco Sauce, Creamy Dreamy Tahini Sauce, Thai Peanut or Almond Sauce, Angry Sauce, Nomato Sauce, Pestos, Four-Flavor Mint Chutney*

NUTS AND SEEDS: *Cashew Sour Cream and Cheeses*

DESSERTS: *Balsamic Reduction*

BREAKFASTS: *Carrot-Tahini Butter, Hippysauce Toast Spread*

FOLLOW YOUR HEART DIP OR SPREAD

Keep the number of ingredients to a minimum as you get started, and let region guide your ingredient combinations.

Combine any combination of:
cooked vegetables, beans, nuts, or seeds

Purée in a food processor with any of the following:
olive oil
sautéed mirepoix (onion, celery, garlic, carrot)
caramelized onions
sautéed mushrooms
roasted garlic, or raw
fresh herbs
lemon or vinegar
salt, tamari, or miso
roasted peppers
olives or capers
sun-dried tomatoes
Cashew Sour Cream (Nuts and Seeds)

Note
- See Menu Planning for notes about combining ingredients to create a cohesive flavor.

Omnivorous variations
- Dairy products like organic yogurt, cream cheese, sour cream, mayonnaise, and melted cheeses are also great bases for dips.

MHAMMARA RED BELL WALNUT DIP

Yields about 1½ cups

Serve this savory Middle Eastern pepper spread as a dip for raw vegetables or bread. You can buy pomegranate molasses at Middle Eastern markets, or substitute as directed below.

Combine and allow to marinate for 5–10 minutes:

1 clove garlic, finely grated

¾ tsp salt

1 Tbsp balsamic vinegar

juice of ½ lemon

Transfer to a food processor with:

1 cup walnuts, toasted (see SPECIAL TECHNIQUES)

Process to grind nuts, then add:

1 lb roasted red bell peppers (about 3) or 1 cup roasted pepper flesh (see SPECIAL TECHNIQUES)

¼ tsp cayenne

¼ tsp cumin

1 tsp smoked paprika

several twists freshly ground black pepper

1 Tbsp pomegranate molasses*

Adjust salt and seasonings to taste.

*To replace pomegranate molasses, use ½ tsp maple syrup and an extra splash of balsamic vinegar or lemon.

Romesco Sauce variation

- To make a version of this Spanish sauce, add roasted tomatoes and a bit of olive oil. Serve over pasta, polenta, or vegetables, or stir into a stew for a flavor blast.

The "secret" to these dips is in the flavor of the raw garlic. When you macerate garlic with acid and salt, the sharp flavor mellows and becomes sweet and refined (see SPECIAL TECHNIQUES).

SECRET GUACAMOLE

Yields about 1 cup

Why would you need a recipe for guacamole? You probably don't, but people often ask why mine is so good. The treatment of the raw garlic makes the difference that your guests will notice.

Combine and allow to briefly marinate:

1 clove garlic, finely grated

2 Tbsp lime juice

½ tsp salt

After 5–10 minutes, add:

1–3 jalapeños, seeded and diced

2 avocados

¼ bunch cilantro, chopped

Mash with a fork, and adjust salt and lime to taste.

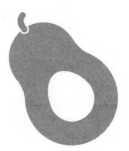

SECRET HUMMUS

....

Yields about 2 cups

This is so delectable when still warm and drizzled with extra olive oil. Use canned beans for a quicker preparation.

Prepare *Home-Cooked Chickpeas for Hummus* (LEGUMES).

Combine and allow to briefly marinate:
  1 clove garlic, finely grated
  juice of 1 lemon
  ¾ tsp salt

After 5–10 minutes, transfer to a food processor with:
2 cups *Home-Cooked Chickpeas for Hummus* (I always include the kombu from cooking the beans, for added minerals)
  ¼ cup + 1 Tbsp tahini
  1 Tbsp tamari or shoyu
  1½ tsp cumin
  ¼ tsp black pepper

Begin processing and slowly drizzle:
  ½ cup olive oil

Add a little water from cooking the beans as needed to make a very creamy texture. Adjust salt and lemon to taste, then add and purée a moment longer to combine well:
  ½ bunch parsley, finely chopped

Variations
  • You can make raw hummus by substituting soaked raw almonds or sunflower seeds for the beans. I like a combination of both.
  • Add kalamata olives, sun-dried tomatoes, roasted red peppers, or other fresh herbs such as cilantro, basil, or chives.

OLIVE-PECAN TAPENADE WITH POMEGRANATE

....

Yields about 1 cup

My friend Jeanne wowed us at a holiday potluck with a tapenade like this. Hers uses walnuts, but I wanted to mix it up, since I already offered a walnut dip. Both are equally outstanding.

Combine in a food processor:

1 clove garlic, finely grated

1 jalapeño, seeded

½ cup extra virgin olive oil

zest of ½ lemon and a squeeze of the juice

Process well, then add:

½ cup pecans or walnuts, or a combination, toasted

1 cup pitted kalamata olives

⅛ tsp black pepper

Process briefly to keep chunky. Stir in:

3 Tbsp chopped Italian parsley

Seeds from ½ pomegranate (see SPECIAL TECHNIQUES)

Note

- If pomegranates are out of season, just omit them or substitute a few dried, chopped figs.

ROASTED GARLIC BABA GHANOUSH

Yields almost 4 cups

See SPECIAL TECHNIQUES to learn how to choose eggplants with fewer seeds. Roast the garlic alongside the eggplant if you use the oven.

Prick with a fork and grill, or preheat oven to 400°:

    2 large eggplants (about 2 lb)

If using oven, roast for about 40 minutes, until thoroughly cooked. Cut in half while still warm and scoop out flesh (should be about 2½ cups). Discard most of the skin, but reserve some for the charred flavor.

Combine in a food processor:

    1 bulb roasted garlic (see SPECIAL TECHNIQUES)

    juice of 1 lemon

    1½ tsp salt

    2 ½ cups cooked eggplant flesh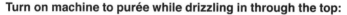

    ¼ cup tahini

    ¼ tsp ground pepper

    1½ tsp cumin

    ⅛ tsp cayenne

    1 tsp smoked paprika

Turn on machine to purée while drizzling in through the top:

    ¼ cup olive oil

Adjust lemon, salt, and spices to taste.

Optional additions

- fresh parsley, mint or cilantro
- olives or fried capers
- roasted red bell peppers or tomatoes

Omnivorous variation

- You may substitute organic yogurt for all or some of the olive oil.

HOMESTEADER'S HONEY MUSTARD

Yields about 1 cup

Many commercial mustards contain unnecessary, unnatural ingredients, but making your own is so easy! This turns out like a nice stone-ground variety, unless your blender is very powerful. Omit the honey if you want a plain, versatile mustard.

Cover with water:

1 Tbsp black mustard seeds

3 Tbsp yellow mustard seeds

½ tsp salt

Soak for 24 hours. Drain, rinse, and place in a blender with:

2 tsp salt

¼ cup honey (optional)

¼ cup apple cider vinegar

¼ cup water

pinch allspice

Blend well, adding a small amount of water if necessary to purée. Allow to mellow for 48 hours before using.

Soups

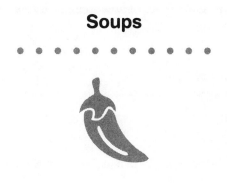

One cannot think well, love well, sleep well, if one has not dined well.

— VIRGINIA WOOLF

Most of my soup recipes are simpler than they might seem. Read through the recipe before you begin so you become familiar with the process and notice how you can multitask along the way. Please read about deglazing in ESSENTIAL TECHNIQUES—most of these recipes refer to it.

To make your soups more nutritious and flavorful, use broth rather than water. Broth is very easy to make from the trimmings of the vegetables you use for the soup. I give a few recipes with a suggested broth, but beware the ingredients of commercial broths and concentrated stock cubes (see ABOUT QUALITY INGREDIENTS). Use water if you must; these soups will still be delicious!

Two more soup recipes in this book are variations of *Smoky Black Bean Chili* (LEGUMES): Smoky Black Bean Soup and Smoky Butternut Squash Soup.

FOLLOW YOUR HEART SOUP

This is a general formula to learn how to make a full-bodied vegan soup out of any ingredients you have available.

Place in a medium soup pot:

1 Tbsp oil

1 onion, diced

¼ tsp salt

Cook over medium-low heat 10–15 minutes, until onions are very soft and translucent. Add:

aromatics (suggest 1 celery, 1 carrot, 2 cloves garlic)

½–1 tsp salt

This base for most soups is called a *mirepoix*. Cook over medium heat for about 5 minutes more, then add:

½ cup wine, tomatoes, fruit or vegetable juice, broth, beer, or water

Deglaze the pan (see ESSENTIAL TECHNIQUES), then let simmer about 7 minutes until nearly dry, taking care to avoid scorching. Add:

4–6 cups vegetable broth or water

additional vegetables, beans, grains, etc.

Bring to a boil, then simmer (partially covered) until thoroughly cooked. Purée if desired, then taste and adjust salt.

Notes

- If the soup still needs something, try a little lemon or vinegar.
- If using miso, stir it in after removing the soup from heat.

Omnivorous variations

- Use butter to sauté onion.
- Use bone broth or milk in place of vegetable broth or water.
- Finish with a little cream after removing from heat.

Additional soup-making tips

- If you need to pause, you can turn off the heat anywhere along the way at the end of a step, before adding the next ingredient.
- If using mushrooms, I usually add them before the ½ cup of liquid, after the mirepoix has had a few minutes to soften.
- When using crushed red pepper flakes or dried Italian seasonings, add them with the mirepoix to soften them and draw out their flavor.
- Use plenty of fat (oil, butter, etc.) to coat the onions and carry the flavors of the aromatics throughout the soup.
- Prior to deglazing, you can use salt as a tool to draw moisture from the onions or vegetables if they start to get dry. You want enough liquid to keep them from burning but not so much that they steam rather than caramelize. If the pan gets too dry, add a little salt, oil, or a tiny bit of water or broth. Or, if you think you've drawn all the sweetness out of the aromatics, perhaps it's time to deglaze.
- When blending puréed soups, place a towel over the top of the blender to protect yourself from splattering.
- While you could just boil all the ingredients at the same time, your soup will be much richer and more complex if you take the time to slowly cook the onions and other aromatics thoroughly first.
- See MENU PLANNING for notes about combining ingredients to create a cohesive flavor.

FOLLOW YOUR HEART VEGETABLE BROTH

The choice of liquid you use in your soup presents an opportunity to increase the nutrients of your meal, not to mention the flavor. Be wary of commercial broths and concentrated stock cubes; they often contain yeast extract or other variations of chemical MSG (see ABOUT QUALITY INGREDIENTS), and are usually very high in sodium as well.

Combine in a large stock pot:

> vegetable scraps such as stems of herbs, tomatoes, mushrooms, seeds and peels from squash or peppers, lettuce, potato peels, and corn-cobs
>
> 1–2 onions, quartered
>
> 2–3 carrots, roughly chopped
>
> 3–4 celery stalks, roughly chopped
>
> 3–4 cloves garlic, smashed
>
> 1 stick kombu seaweed, whole
>
> 1–2 bay leaves
>
> 1 tsp black peppercorns
>
> 8 cups water

Bring to a boil, then simmer for 20–40 minutes, partially covered. Strain.

Additional broth-making notes

- All of the ingredients listed are optional. Vegetable broth is very flexible and leaves plenty of room for creativity. Be modest with strong flavors, but you may want to select ingredients to enhance the flavor of the soup you are making.
- Use any clean vegetable scraps that still have life in them, except those noted below. Fresh herbs are nice additions, but dried herbs can easily overpower the broth, so use them sparingly.
- Avoid cruciferous or overpowering vegetables such as cabbage, broccoli, cauliflower, and beets.
- To intensify the flavor, you can caramelize the vegetables first by cooking them with oil in the pot or a hot oven prior to covering them with water.

- If you don't salt your broth, you can more easily control the saltiness of your soups.
- You can also use broth instead of water to cook grains to increase their flavor and nutrition.
- Freeze broth in small containers so you always have some on hand for a quick soup.

A NOTE ABOUT ANIMAL BONE BROTHS

Homemade bone broths are tremendously nourishing and replenishing, and make use of the parts of animals that are often wastefully discarded. Vegetarians who discover that they need animal-based nutrition in their diets may find that using bone broth in soups or to cook grains is more palatable than eating meat. These broths need to cook at least 3–4 hours, with a dash of vinegar to help draw out the nutrients.

"Itadakimasu" is Japanese meal blessing that means "I humbly receive." It is meant to acknowledge and express gratitude to all who played a role in preparing, cultivating, hunting, or sacrificing life for the meal.

SIMPLE SILKY ZUCCHINI SOUP

Yields 4–6 servings

This soup is so simple and easy. The garnishes are optional but can take the soup in any number of directions. Thanks to San Francisco chef Orchid for the inspiration.

Place in a medium soup pot:

1 Tbsp olive oil

1 yellow onion, diced

¼ tsp salt

Cook over medium-low heat for 7 minutes, then add:

1 small potato, diced

Sauté about 5 more minutes, until onions are translucent. Add:

1½ lb zucchini (about 6), roughly chopped

2 Tbsp fresh herbs (oregano, marjoram, thyme, etc.), minced

¾ tsp salt

Cook 5 minutes more until garlic is fragrant and squash is seared. Add:

¼ cup white wine

Deglaze bottom of pot (see Essential Techniques) and simmer about 7 minutes until nearly dry again. Add:

4 cups water or vegetable broth

Bring to a boil, reduce heat, and simmer for 10 minutes, until squash is well cooked. Purée with:

½ tsp salt, to taste

1 Tbsp lemon juice

Garnish suggestions

- Swirl in a *Pesto* (Sauces) or pistou, a bit of quality olive oil, or a dollop of *Cashew Sour Cream* (Nuts and Seeds).
- Add chopped capers, olives, or fresh herbs.
- Try cherry tomatoes sautéed with garlic and parsley.

Carrot-Ginger Soup variation

- Replace zucchini with carrots, and herbs with grated fresh ginger. You may enjoy lime in place of lemon to complement the Asian flavors of this soup.

Omnivorous variations

- You may substitute butter in place of oil to sauté the vegetables.
- You may substitute bone broth in place of vegetable broth or water.
- Garnish with a dollop of yogurt, butter, or heavy cream before serving.

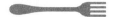

CHILLED CUCUMBER MINT SOUP

Yields 3 cups

This light soup makes a bright start to a hearty summer meal, and is very refreshing by the cupful on a hot afternoon.

Purée in blender:

3 cucumbers, peeled

1 tsp salt

3 Tbsp lime juice

¼ cup mint leaves, packed

2–3 Tbsp olive oil

Adjust lime and salt to taste.

SUMMER'S GLORY GAZPACHO

Yields 3 cups

Use tomatoes at the height of their season for this delightful soup. If you are using less-than-perfect tomatoes, roast them first to bring out their sweetness. This recipe is worth splurging on a high-quality, fruity olive oil.

Combine in a blender:

¼ cup red onion, chopped

3 Tbsp lime juice

1 jalapeño chile, seeded and chopped

½ tsp cumin powder

¼ cup packed fresh cilantro

2 lb fresh in-season tomatoes (about 5 medium)

few grinds black pepper

1 sprig fresh oregano leaves

1½ -2 tsp salt, to taste

1 small red bell pepper (optional)

Begin to purée, while SLOWLY drizzling:

⅓ cup quality olive oil

Adjust lime and salt to taste. Serve chilled.

WHITE BEAN SOUP WITH KALE

Yields 4–6 servings

Presoaked beans cook in this soup to make a rich broth. Serve with crusty bread or a pilaf (GRAINS) for a complete meal.

Combine in a large soup pot:

1 Tbsp olive oil

1 large yellow onion, diced

Cook over medium-low heat about 15 minutes, until onions are well cooked. Add:

1 rib celery, diced

1 carrot, diced

3–4 cloves garlic, minced

Continue to cook for 3–5 minutes, until garlic is fragrant. Add:

½ cup white wine

Deglaze bottom of pot (see ESSENTIAL TECHNIQUES) and simmer briefly. Add:

1½ cups white beans, soaked overnight

1 sprig rosemary and 5 sprigs thyme, tied with a string

6 cups water

Bring to a boil, then simmer until beans are soft, a little over an hour. Remove herb stems and add:

½ bunch kale, chopped

1½ tsp salt

½ tsp black pepper

½ cup puréed tomatoes

Simmer 3–4 more minutes, until kale is cooked. Add:

squeeze of lemon juice

salt, to taste

Omnivorous variation

- You can substitute butter in place of oil to sauté the vegetables.

COCONUT MASOOR DAHL

Yields 4–5 servings

This hearty soup is spicy and deeply flavorful. It stands well alone or as a starting course in an Indian-themed meal.

Place in a soup pot:

1 Tbsp coconut oil

1 yellow onion, diced

1 tsp salt

Cook over medium heat about 10 minutes, until onions are translucent.

Add:

2 garlic cloves, minced

1 Tbsp minced or grated ginger

1–2 serrano or jalapeño peppers, seeded and diced small

Cook for another 5 minutes, then add:

½ tsp cumin

½ tsp coriander

2 tsp mustard seeds, toasted separately until popping

½ tsp turmeric

¼ tsp cayenne or crushed red pepper flakes (optional)

Cook a few minutes more, until spices are fragrant.

Add:

½ cup tomatoes or white wine

Deglaze pan (see Essential Techniques) then add:

1 cup red lentils

2½ cups water or broth

Bring to a boil, then turn down heat to simmer about 20–30 minutes, until lentils are well cooked. Stir often and add a little water if lentils are sticking before they're soft. Add:

1 cup coconut milk

juice of 1 lime

Adjust salt and lime to taste.

Garnish suggestions

- cilantro, chopped
- lime wedges
- onion, minced and marinated briefly in lime juice
- toasted dried coconut

> *Cooking creates a sense of well-being for yourself and the people you love, and brings beauty and meaning to everyday life. And all it requires is common sense— the common sense to eat seasonally, to know where your food comes from, to support and buy from local farmers and producers who are good stewards of our natural resources.*
>
> — ALICE WATERS

HEALING HOT AND SOUR SOUP
....

Yields 4–5 servings

This soup makes a comforting meal for the sick when chicken soup won't do. I garnish it with as much cilantro as they can stand—it's very purifying.

Start a broth (optional, see end of recipe).

Combine in a small bowl to make miso base and set aside:

¼ cup miso (dissolve in a little broth or water first)

1 tsp toasted sesame oil

1 Tbsp tamari or shoyu

1–2 Tbsp brown rice vinegar, to taste

¼–½ tsp white pepper, to taste

Combine in a large heavy soup pot:

1 Tbsp olive or light sesame oil

1 leek, white and light green parts only, sliced thinly

¼ tsp salt

Cover and cook over medium heat, stirring occasionally, until leeks wilt and begin to stick (about 8–10 minutes). Add:

1 carrot, cut into matchsticks (see SPECIAL TECHNIQUES)

2–3 large cloves garlic, minced

Stir and cover again. Cook about 3 more minutes, then add:

½ cup apple juice

few large pinches crushed red pepper, to taste

Deglaze pan (see ESSENTIAL TECHNIQUES) and simmer about 5 minutes, until nearly dry again. Add:

½ cup shredded cabbage or kale

¼ cup wakame

6 cups hot broth or water

1–3 tsp grated fresh ginger, to taste

Simmer about 5 minutes, until greens are cooked. Add:

miso base, above

Adjust seasonings to taste.

Garnish suggestions

- scallions, thinly sliced
- cilantro, leaves and stems finely chopped
- mung bean sprouts
- *Savory Roasted Shiitakes* (ROASTIES)
- *Gomasio Salt* (NUTS AND SEEDS)

Broth suggestions

leek greens

1 carrot

2 cloves garlic, smashed

1-inch piece ginger, roughly chopped

stems from ½ bunch cilantro

1 Tbsp black peppercorns

1–2 strips of kombu seaweed

6 cups water

Bring to a boil, then simmer, partially covered, until you are ready to strain and use in soup.

ROASTED CORN CHOWDER WITH POBLANO CHILES

Yields 4–5 servings

The vegetable parings here are especially flavorful, so I always make a broth while I prepare this soup (see end of recipe).

Combine in large, wide baking dish:

¾ lb Yukon Gold or red potatoes (about 3), diced small

2½ cups corn kernels (about 3 ears)

¼ tsp ground cumin

½ tsp chili powder

generous drizzle olive oil

½ tsp salt

Roast at about 450°, stirring occasionally, about 20–30 minutes.

Roast, peel, and dice according to instructions for red bell peppers in SPECIAL TECHNIQUES:

¾ lb poblano chiles, whole (about 3) or pasilla, ancho, or anaheim chiles

Combine in a large soup pot:

1 Tbsp olive oil

1 yellow onion, diced

1 medium carrot, cut into rounds

1 large stalk celery, sliced

¼ tsp salt

Cook over medium-low heat about 10 minutes, until onions begin to color. Add:

1 large clove garlic, minced

½ tsp chili powder

Cook for about 3 minutes, until garlic is fragrant. Add:

½ cup white wine

Deglaze pan (see ESSENTIAL TECHNIQUES**) and simmer about 5 minutes, until nearly dry again. Add:**

roasted potatoes, corn, and chiles, above

Stir and cook for about 2 more minutes, until nearly dry. Add:

4 cups broth or water

¼–½ tsp salt

Simmer 10 minutes. Remove 2 cups to a blender with:

1 cup *Nut Mylk* (NUTS AND SEEDS)

Blend briefly and stir back into soup. Adjust seasonings to taste.

Garnish suggestions

- black pepper
- chopped cilantro and scallions
- *Cashew Sour Cream* (NUTS AND SEEDS)
- 1 fresh red bell pepper, diced small

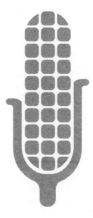

Broth suggestions

1 onion, plus parings from recipe

corn cobs and potato parings

2 cloves garlic, smashed

seeds from roasted chiles

stems from 1 bunch cilantro

1 Tbsp black peppercorns

1–2 strips of kombu seaweed

4 cups water

Bring to a boil, then simmer, partially covered, until you are ready to strain and use in soup.

Omnivorous variations

- You may substitute butter in place of oil to sauté the onions, carrots, and celery.
- You may substitute bone broth in place of vegetable broth or water.
- You may substitute milk or cream for the *Nut Mylk*.
- Garnish with a dollop of yogurt, sour cream, butter, or heavy cream before serving.

ANGRY CAULIFLOWER POTAGE

Yields 6–8 servings

This easy soup is a cross between *Angry Sauce* and *Spicy Roasted Cauliflower.* The entire process uses only the oven, then the blender.

Preheat oven to 425°.

Combine in a large casserole dish:

2 lb Roma tomatoes, quartered or smaller

1 medium head cauliflower, cut into large florets

1 red onion, chopped

2 red bell peppers, chopped (optional)

5 large cloves garlic, chopped

½–1 tsp crushed red pepper, to taste

2–3 Tbsp olive oil

1 tsp salt

freshly ground pepper

1–2 sprigs fresh rosemary, chopped

Roast for about 30 minutes until cauliflower is cooked, stirring every 10 minutes or so. Add:

dash of balsamic vinegar or lemon juice

Purée in batches in a blender with:

5–6 cups vegetable broth or water

Use enough liquid to create the creamy consistency to your liking. Adjust salt, pepper, and vinegar or lemon to taste. Garnish with:

drizzle of a quality olive oil

fresh herbs, minced (parsley, oregano, thyme, basil, etc.)

Roasties

· · · · · · · · · · · ·

**When faced with an unfamiliar vegetable, toss it with
olive oil and salt, then roast it in a hot oven until it is
soft. It will probably be good to eat.**

Roasties are so simple and delicious that they are regulars at my table.
I serve them as side dishes, taco fillings, and even savory breakfasts in
place of home fries. They're a great accompaniment to non-vegetarian
meals to encourage your family to eat more vegetables. I use a fairly hot,
preheated oven (400°–425°) to caramelize the sugars in the vegetables,
but the temperature is not necessarily important, so you can roast alongside other recipes that are more temperature-sensitive.

Stir your veggies occasionally while roasting, and change the pan's posi-
tion if the heat is distributing unevenly. Give them plenty of space so they
don't steam; you want the moisture to evaporate so the sugars caramelize.
I always salt veggies lightly before roasting and again just before serving
to heighten the flavor.

If you use different vegetables in the same pan, be sure to cut them into
sizes that will ensure even cooking. Cut denser, longer-cooking vegetables
(like root vegetables or winter squash) into smaller pieces than softer,
faster-cooking ones (such as mushrooms or summer squash).

GOOD CANDIDATES FOR ROASTING

Artichoke

Asparagus

Brussels sprouts

Cauliflower

Chile peppers and sweet peppers

Eggplant (see notes in SPECIAL TECHNIQUES)

Fennel, endive, and radicchio bulbs

Garlic (see SPECIAL TECHNIQUES)

Mushrooms (shiitake, portobello, cremini, etc.)

Onions

Leeks and scallions

Roots of all kinds (potatoes, beets, parsnips, turnips, rutabaga, sweet potatoes, carrots, etc.)

Summer squash (zucchini, pattypan, etc.)

Tomatoes

Winter squash (butternut, delicata, kabocha, etc.)

Note

- Vegetables may be left whole or cut evenly into any size. If you are combining vegetables, cut the denser, longer-cooking ones smaller than those that cook faster.

ROASTED ROOT MEDLEY

Yields 4 servings

The lemon is a nice surprise in this basic roasted vegetable dish. Be sure to cut longer-cooking vegetables into smaller pieces than those that cook faster. Serve with grains or pasta, and top with a sauce if desired.

Preheat oven to about 425°. Combine in an ovenproof dish:

2 lb assorted root vegetables, evenly chopped

2 Tbsp olive oil

1 tsp salt, to taste

2 cloves garlic, chopped

1 lemon, sliced into rounds (scrubbed and unpeeled)

1 sprig fresh rosemary, minced

Roast at about 425° until soft (usually anywhere from 20 to 50 minutes, depending on size and density of vegetables). Stir once or twice during cooking, and season again with a little salt before serving.

Leftovers

- Extra roasties are handy to have on hand to add to breakfast scrambles, salads, burritos, tacos, or perhaps a *Follow Your Heart Dip.*

Omnivorous variation

- Roasties are a great side dish for nonvegetarian meals. They can also be added to frittatas, omelets, quiches, or scrambled eggs.

SAVORY ROASTED SHIITAKES

Easy, meaty, delicious, and nutritious, these are among my favorite foods ever. Serve these roasted mushrooms whole as a snack or side dish, or add to sushi, soups, or pasta.

Preheat oven to 400° (the exact temperature isn't crucial).

Combine in an ovenproof dish:

fresh shiitake mushrooms, left whole

salt, to taste

drizzle of olive oil to coat

dash of water

Place mushrooms stem-side down and roast for 10 minutes. Turn each mushroom over and continue to cook about 5–10 minutes more, until stems are cooked through. Sprinkle lightly with a touch more salt before serving.

Notes

- Select mushrooms that are large, moist, and evenly sized, or pull out the smaller, faster-cooking ones as they are finished so as not to overcook them.
- If the stems are particularly thick or woody, slice them in half or even quarters so they cook thoroughly. The stems are the most nutritious part so be sure to cook them well.

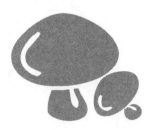

BALSAMIC GLAZED BEETS

These next three recipes demonstrate a simple way to add variety to ROAS-TIES by adding a sauce or glaze toward the end of cooking. Serve these scrumptious beets with salads, as a side dish, or even on pizza. Add thick slices of red onion if you like.

Preheat oven to about 400°.

Combine in an ovenproof dish:

6 beets, peeled and cut into large chunks

2 Tbsp olive oil, to coat

1 tsp salt

Roast until almost completely cooked through, up to 45 minutes. Drizzle with:

3 Tbsp balsamic vinegar

1 Tbsp maple syrup

¼–½ tsp salt, to taste

Return to oven until somewhat dry, up to 10 minutes. (Stir once or twice to distribute glaze.) Adjust salt and finish with freshly ground pepper.

Balsamic Glazed Figs variation

- Substitute fresh, whole figs for beets. Cook only 15–20 minutes. These are delicious for dessert over vanilla ice cream.

Orange Glazed Asparagus or Fennel variation

- Substitute asparagus spears or large slices of fennel for the beets and orange juice for the balsamic. Finish with a sprinkle of orange zest.

Omnivorous variation

- Organic feta cheese is a nice complement to these beets.

CREAMY TAHINI-COATED ROASTIES
....

Yields 6 servings

Winter squash, cauliflower, onions, and roots such as carrots, beets, turnips, and parsnips are my favorite vegetables for this preparation.

Prepare:

Roasted Root Medley, using the vegetables of your choice (omit rosemary)

Moments before vegetables are fully cooked, stir in a sauce made of:

¼ cup tahini

1 Tbsp rice vinegar

1 Tbsp tamari

2–4 Tbsp water, to achieve a pourable consistency

Return to oven for 3–5 more minutes to allow the sauce to dry a bit and get sticky.

Stovetop method

- Sauté mixed vegetables and add the tahini sauce above when they're almost fully cooked. Stir and continue cooking 3–5 minutes more until sauce has become sticky and vegetables are thoroughly cooked. This stovetop method is great for cabbage, broccoli, carrots, onion, and cauliflower.

SPICY ROASTED CAULIFLOWER

Yields 4–6 servings

This is inspired by a side dish at one of my favorite Italian bistros in San Francisco, Delfina Pizzeria. Roasted cauliflower has an unexpected sweetness and nice caramelized texture.

Preheat oven to about 450°.

Combine:

    1 medium head cauliflower, cut into large florets

    1 large tomato, peeled and diced (see SPECIAL TECHNIQUES)

    2–3 Tbsp capers, rinsed

    ½–1 tsp salt

    ½–1 tsp crushed red pepper, to taste

    6–8 cloves garlic, to taste

    4–6 Tbsp olive oil, to coat generously

Arrange in a single layer on baking sheets. Roast for 20–30 minutes, until cauliflower is tender and golden brown, stirring every 10 minutes or so. Adjust salt and freshly ground pepper to taste. Garnish with:

    minced parsley

    Nut Parm (NUTS AND SEEDS)

Note

- While the temperature is flexible, a high temperature makes the cauliflower crispier and more caramelized.

Omnivorous variation

- Substitute grated organic Parmesan cheese for the *Nut Parm*.

MISO-GLAZED JAPANESE EGGPLANT

Yields 4–6 servings

This recipe is awesome with rice or noodles. It will win over even a die-hard eggplant aversion, but the sauce is also great with other vegetables or tofu substituted.

Preheat oven to about 400°.

Combine in a small bowl:

2 Tbsp miso

1–2 tsp honey or other syrup

2 tsp sesame oil

1 Tbsp rice vinegar

1 Tbsp grated fresh ginger

2 cloves garlic, finely grated

3 Tbsp water

pinch crushed red pepper flakes (optional)

Set this sauce aside.

Combine in a baking dish:

4 Japanese eggplants, cut into large diagonal chunks or sliced in half
    lengthwise

olive oil, to coat

¼ tsp salt

Roast for about 25 minutes, then stir in sauce (above) and return to oven for 5–8 minutes more. Garnish with:

Gomasio Salt (NUTS AND SEEDS) or toasted walnuts

scallions, sliced thin on the diagonal

Omnivorous variation

• You may also want to try this sweet miso glaze with fish.

Vegetables

Eat food. Not too much. Mostly plants.

—MICHAEL POLLAN

I usually serve vegetables very simply: lightly sautéed, roasted, or steamed, with some grains or beans and a sauce—or any combination thereof. Most of the recipes in this book include vegetables, so the recipes in this chapter are just a few of my favorite vegetable-based preparations.

Use these recipes as-is for vegan or vegetarian diets, or alongside non-vegetarian meals to encourage your family to eat more vegetables. Enjoy!

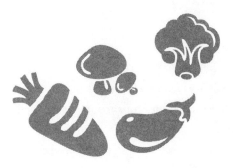

FOLLOW YOUR HEART ENCHILADAS

Yields 12 enchiladas

This traditional method of dipping the tortillas in hot oil makes for a full-bodied flavor, and keeps the tortillas from falling apart.

Prepare:

3 cups of a flavorful filling, suggestions below

and:

2 cups of sauce, either *Fresh Tomatillo Salsa Verde* or *Kipahulu Taco Sauce* (SAUCES)

Pour 1 cup sauce into a wide baking dish and set the rest aside.

Preheat oven to 350°. Warm gently in a wide skillet:

3 Tbsp oil

When the oil is barely shimmering from the heat, place into pan, several at a time:

12 organic corn tortillas

Cook each tortilla just enough to soften, 10–20 seconds, then remove with tongs and drain on paper towels. Roll about ¼ cup of prepared filling into each tortilla and arrange in baking dish. Pour remaining cup of sauce over enchiladas, cover, and bake for 25 minutes. Garnish with:

Cashew Sour Cream (NUTS AND SEEDS)

Secret Guacamole (DIPS AND SPREADS)

Tamari-Toasted Seeds (NUTS AND SEEDS)

red onion and cilantro, chopped

Filling suggestions

- *Smoky Black Bean Chili* (LEGUMES)
- *Tempeh Apple Sausage Hash* (BREAKFASTS)
- black beans with corn and mushrooms, seasoned with onions and chili powder
- sweet potatoes or butternut squash, cooked with orange juice, garlic, and chipotle powder

- sautéed zucchini, potatoes, and onions, seasoned with cumin
- pinto beans and rice with sautéed or roasted poblano chiles

Omnivorous variations

- Add organic cheese or meat to the filling, and top with cheese or sour cream.

> *Any scientist who tells you they know that GMOs are safe and not to worry about it, is either ignorant of the history of science or is deliberately lying. Nobody knows what the long-term effect will be.*
>
> — DAVID SUZUKI, GENETICIST

RAW ZUCCHINI PASTA
....

Yields 4 servings

If you want to get serious about making raw pasta, it's fun to get a spiralizer, which makes long thin spaghetti strips out of vegetables such as zucchini or butternut squash. Find them at Asian markets or online.

Combine in a small bowl to make the sauce:

½ red onion, thinly sliced

1 clove garlic, finely grated

½ tsp salt

1 Tbsp lemon juice

2–3 Tbsp balsamic vinegar (just enough to cover onions)

Set aside to marinate while you prepare other ingredients.

Combine in a large bowl:

8 large *Savory Roasted Shiitakes* (Roasties), sliced thickly

2 Tbsp kalamata olives, chopped, or 1 Tbsp capers, rinsed

½ cup cherry or sun-dried tomatoes, sliced

up to ½ cup fresh Italian herbs, minced—basil, oregano, parsley, etc.

salt and freshly ground pepper, to taste

Toss with sauce (above) and:

4 medium zucchinis, shredded, thinly sliced, or spiralized

3–4 Tbsp quality olive oil

Serve on a bed of salad greens and garnish with:

2–4 Tbsp *Nut Parm* (Nuts and Seeds)

¼ tsp crushed red pepper flakes

Variation

- This recipe is equally delicious with regular cooked pasta instead of zucchini "noodles."
- Raw pasta is also excellent with the Creamy Pasta Sauce variation of *Cashew Hollandaise* (Breakfasts).

Omnivorous variation

- Substitute freshly shredded organic Parmesan cheese for the *Nut Parm.*

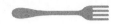

MARVELOUS MUSHROOMS WITH WINE AND HERBS

Yields 4 servings

This succulent side dish will make your house smell delicious! I always use creminis or portobello mushrooms, and any wild mushrooms available. This recipe also makes a nice accompaniment for pasta with extra wine and oil.

Combine in a medium pan:

1½ lb mushrooms, stems removed

pinch crushed red pepper flakes (optional)

2 Tbsp olive oil

Sauté 10 minutes over medium heat. Add:

4 cloves garlic, minced

2 Tbsp Italian parsley, minced

1 Tbsp tomato paste (optional)

¼ cup dry white wine

Sauté about 4 minutes, gradually turning up the heat to simmer until liquid reduces. Season with:

1 Tbsp fresh herbs (thyme, marjoram, basil, etc.)

2 Tbsp chives or scallion tops, chopped

salt and pepper, to taste

Cook 1 more minute to incorporate flavors.

Omnivorous variation

- Substitute butter for olive oil.

THAI GREEN CURRY VEGETABLE STEW

Yields about 4 servings

Delicious and easy, this is great over *Coconut Jasmine Rice* (GRAINS). Choose a quality curry paste with all-natural ingredients (see ABOUT QUALITY INGREDIENTS).

Combine in a medium soup pot:

1 Tbsp coconut oil

1 yellow or white onion, diced

1 tsp salt

Cook over medium heat for about 8–10 minutes, until onion is translucent. Add:

1 Tbsp grated fresh ginger

2 cloves garlic, minced

1–3 Tbsp prepared Thai green curry paste

¼ cup mirin, white wine, stock, or water

Cook for 3 minutes more, stirring to lift pieces off the bottom of pan. Add:

4 cups assorted vegetables, such as zucchini, broccoli, bell peppers, mushrooms, and snow peas

1 can full-fat coconut milk

Simmer until vegetables are cooked. Add:

¼ cup whole Thai basil leaves

juice of 1 lime

1–2 tsp Sucanat or coconut sugar, to taste

Adjust salt, sweetener, and lime to taste. Serve over rice.

Variation

- To add protein to this dish, add tofu (fresh or fried separately in coconut oil) with the seasoned coconut milk. Simmer until almost fully cooked before adding vegetables so as not to overcook them.
- I sometimes blanch and shock (see ESSENTIAL TECHNIQUES) the

vegetables separately and add them at the end to keep them perfectly cooked.

Omnivorous variation

- If you want animal protein with this vegan stew, simmer pieces of organic, pasture-raised meat, chicken, or fish in the seasoned coconut milk until almost fully cooked before adding vegetables so as not to overcook them.

SWEET AND SOUR GLAZED VEGETABLES

Yields 4 servings

Spicy, sweet, and sour flavors come together in a delicious glaze for all kinds of vegetables. Serve these over rice or noodles, or with fried or braised tempeh.

Combine in a small bowl to make the sauce:

1 Tbsp miso paste

2 Tbsp tamari

2 Tbsp rice vinegar

1½ Tbsp honey

1 Tbsp non-GMO cornstarch or arrowroot

1 Tbsp toasted sesame oil

Stir well to dissolve starch and set aside.

Combine in a large pan:

1 Tbsp coconut oil

¼–½ tsp crushed red pepper, to taste

1 tsp minced garlic

1 tsp minced ginger

2 lb mixed vegetables (onion, carrot, cabbage, cauliflower, broccoli, etc.)

Stir-fry over medium-high heat for 3–6 minutes until vegetables are cooked. Add sauce and cook 1 minute more, until the vegetables are glazed. Salt to taste and garnish with:

4 scallions, thinly sliced on the diagonal

Omnivorous variation

- This vegan recipe is a nice side dish for fish, and you can also use the glaze on the fish itself.

SPICY BBQ POTATO SALAD

Yields 6–8 servings

Yukons and red potatoes hold up best for potato salads. Dress the potatoes while they're still warm so they can absorb the flavors.

Combine in a medium pot:

3 lb potatoes, scrubbed or peeled, diced evenly

2 Tbsp salt

water to cover

Bring to a boil, reduce heat, and simmer 10–15 minutes, until barely tender.

Drain well and toss with a dressing made of:

1 recipe *Creamy Chipotle Dressing* (DRESSINGS)

1 tsp extra salt, to taste

1 Tbsp extra tahini

1 Tbsp extra lemon or vinegar, to taste

Stir in:

2 ribs celery, sliced

½ cup small red onion, diced

1 red bell pepper, diced

1 carrot, shredded or finely diced

½ cup cherry tomatoes, cut in half

Drizzle with:

olive oil

Adjust salt and seasonings to taste.

Variation

- Add pieces of *Tempeh Bacon* (BREAKFASTS).

Omnivorous variation

- If you want animal protein with this vegan potato salad, add pieces of chopped organic pastured bacon.

JAPANESE KINPIRA VEGETABLES

Yields 4–6 servings

Burdock is an awesome liver cleanser, especially important at the onset of spring and fall but always beneficial. I eat this with rice or in sushi, or just alone in a big heap. It looks very pretty served with chopsticks!

Combine in a large, wide pan:

5 carrot-sized burdock roots, cut into matchsticks (see Special Tech-niques)

4 carrots, cut into matchsticks

2 parsnips or turnips, cut into matchsticks

2-inch piece ginger, grated

pinch salt

2 Tbsp light sesame oil, or any light oil

Cook over medium-high heat for 2–3 minutes, then add just enough water to cover the bottom of the skillet—do not cover the vegetables, just the bottom of the pan. Also add:

2 Tbsp rice vinegar or mirin

Cover and cook over medium heat until the vegetables are almost cooked, then add:

2 Tbsp tamari or shoyu

1 Tbsp toasted sesame oil

Stir to combine, cover, and cook 2–3 minutes. Remove the cover and cook off the excess liquid, taking care not to burn the tamari.

Variations

- Add 1–2 Tbsp dried hijiki seaweed with the rice vinegar.
- Stir in a few tablespoons of toasted sesame seeds at the end. (Black seeds are particularly stunning.)

CURTIDO SALAD WITH PEPITAS

Yields 5–6 servings

A roommate from El Salvador taught me this traditional coleslaw, which is usually served with pupusas (thick stuffed, fried tortillas). It's become indispensable to me. I serve it with tacos and most Latin-themed meals.

Combine in a large bowl:

¼ cup apple cider vinegar or lime juice

½ tsp salt

½ tsp sugar (optional)

1 tsp dried oregano, rubbed between palms

¼ red onion, thinly sliced

1 Tbsp olive oil

Add:

½ head green cabbage, shredded

1 carrot, shredded

1 jalapeño, seeded and diced

½ bunch cilantro, chopped

Toss and adjust salt, vinegar and other seasonings to taste. Allow to marinate at least 30 minutes, up to 24 hours.

Garnish with:

¼ cup *Tamari-Toasted Pumpkin Seeds* (NUTS AND SEEDS)

Creamy Coleslaw variation

- To make a vegan old-fashioned creamy slaw, toss cabbage, carrot, and your favorite slaw vegetables with any of the following dressings: *Farmgirl Ranch, Creamy Chipotle, Lemon Tahini,* or *Homesteader's Honey Mustard.*

MASSAGED KALE SALAD

Yields 2–4 servings

I love kale. I eat it every day and thank it for strengthening my bones. I usually chop it very fine, down to the tough bottom of the spine. If you're new to kale, you may want to pull off the tender leaves and discard the spine until you can enjoy its hearty texture.

In a large salad bowl, combine and allow to marinate 5–10 minutes:

1 small clove garlic, finely grated

¾ tsp salt

2–3 Tbsp balsamic vinegar

¼ to ½ cup thinly sliced red onion, to taste

Add and allow to marinate a few minutes more:

1 beet, shredded

Add:

1 bunch kale, finely chopped (see SPECIAL TECHNIQUES)

drizzle of quality olive oil

Using your hands, firmly massage the salad for about 5 minutes until the kale is tenderized.

Add:

¼ cup walnuts, toasted or raw

freshly ground black pepper, to taste

handful of cherry tomatoes or dried cranberries, cut in half (optional)

Toss and serve at once or refrigerate up to 8 hours.

Variations

- Any of the SALAD DRESSINGS are great on raw massaged kale salads.
- To make a really easy raw kale salad, simply massage chopped kale with some *Simple Sauerkraut* or *Spring Tonic Chee* (VEGETABLES). Add avocado and *Tamari Toasted Seeds* (NUTS AND SEEDS) for healthy fats and protein.

RAPINI WITH GARLIC AND LEMON

Yields 2–4 servings

Also called rabe or Chinese broccoli, rapini is a pungent green vegetable with long stalks, sharp leaves, and small florets that resemble broccoli. This side dish is also excellent over pasta with extra garlic and olive oil.

Combine in a pan:

1 Tbsp olive oil

2 cloves garlic, minced

pinch crushed red pepper

Cook for about 1 minute, tossing well to coat with oil. Add:

1 bunch rapini, ¼ inch of stem removed and cut into 2-inch pieces

3 Tbsp water

Stir well, cover, and cook about 7 minutes until tender, stirring occasionally. Add:

juice of ½ lemon, to taste

salt, to taste

Variations

- Add or substitute broccoli, or any variety of chopped kale, bok choy, or mustard greens.
- Add *Savory Roasted Shiitakes* (ROASTIES), a drizzle of tamari, and a few drops of toasted sesame oil.
- Garnish with *Tamari-Toasted Seeds* or *Nut Parm* (NUTS AND SEEDS).

Omnivorous variation

- You may want to garnish this vegan side dish with freshly shredded organic Parmesan cheese.

SIMPLE SAUERKRAUT

Yields 1 gallon

Making your own kraut is very easy and satisfying. It's an inexpensive probiotic digestive aid and a nutritious, zesty addition to a salad, sandwich, or grain bowl. Check out Sandor Katz's website and awesome fermentation books for lots of helpful information about krauts.

Combine:

5 lb cabbage, shredded

3 Tbsp salt

Massage the cabbage with the salt using firm pressure for a couple of minutes, then pack it as tightly as possible into a clean gallon jar, bucket, or ceramic crock.

Place a heavy weight on top to press the cabbage down, such as a jug of water. The salt will continue to break the cabbage down and cause it to release water, creating the brine that will preserve it. Press the cabbage down a few times over the first few days and keep it submerged in the brine with the heavy weight. (Contact with oxygen will make it spoil.)

Cover with a cloth and keep at room temperature for one to five weeks, tasting periodically for the flavor you like. If mold develops on the surface, just skim and discard it; the kraut below is still preserved in the brine. When it has reached the flavor you like, pack into smaller jars and refrigerate it to stop the fermentation process. It will generally keep for up to a year in the refrigerator.

Note

You can add almost any vegetables, greens, seasonings, or fruits to the cabbage. I like to shred or slice each ingredient differently so the end result is varied and interesting. A few suggestions to get you started:

- Apple, onion, and caraway seeds.
- Ginger, cauliflower, and sea vegetables.
- Combination of root vegetables, such as turnips, carrots, and beets.

SPRING TONIC CHEE

Yields 1 gallon

Burdock and dandelion cleanse the liver, which is beneficial at the turns of seasons. Fermentation mellows the medicinal bitterness of dandelion greens. Try this version of kim chee over plain rice with steamed broccoli and *Thai Almond or Peanut Sauce* (SAUCES) or in a raw kale salad.

Combine in a very large bowl, or divide into 2 bowls:

2 heads green cabbage, shredded (about 2½ lb)

1 daikon, sliced into thin circles (about 1 lb)

4 carrots, matchsticks or grated (about ¾ lb)

4 large burdock roots, thinly sliced (about 1 lb)

1 bunch dandelion leaves, thinly sliced

1 yellow onion, thinly sliced

2-inch piece ginger, grated

3 Tbsp salt

Massage with firm pressure for a few minutes, then use tongs or a spoon (to protect fingers from burning) to add:

3 hot chiles, chopped or ½–1 tsp crushed red pepper flakes

Pack firmly into a gallon jar, bucket, or crock and follow instructions for *Simple Sauerkraut*.

Tip

To make the job easier, I combine the vegetables and salt and let them stand for a few hours to break them down a bit before massaging.

Variation

- If you prefer a milder version, omit the dandelion leaves and chiles. The ginger sweetens this combination as it ferments.

MISSION PICKLES

Yields about 25 oz

Named for the *jalapeños en escabeche* served at every taqueria in San Francisco's beloved Mission district. This spicy pickle is the perfect accompaniment to any Latin-inspired meal.

Combine in a small saucepan:

1½ cups water

1½ cups apple cider vinegar

3 jalapeños, sliced lengthwise

5 cloves garlic, peeled and lightly smashed

1½ tsp salt

½ tsp sugar

4 bay leaves

1 tsp cumin seeds

½ tsp dried Mexican oregano

¼ tsp whole peppercorns

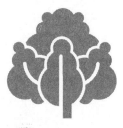

Bring to a boil, then reduce heat and simmer for 10 minutes.

Add:

1 lb carrots (4–6), peeled and sliced ¼ inch on the bias

½ yellow onion, sliced

Simmer until cooked (5–10 minutes), then allow to cool in the brine overnight. Place in a jar with a tight lid and keep refrigerated up to 3 weeks.

Variations

- Use this method to pickle any variety of vegetables in seasoned vinegar: cucumbers, beets, green beans, radishes, cauliflower, onion, etc.
- Different seasonings can vary the flavors of your pickles, such as coriander, cardamom, allspice, fennel, mustard seeds, dill seeds, and black peppercorns. Experiment and enjoy!

Nuts and Seeds

Nuts and seeds—as well as grains and legumes—are dormant plants, designed to survive the digestive systems of humans and animals. You can make their nutrients more available for digestion by soaking them to induce germination. This process is called sprouting.

Since they are burgeoning new life, sprouts develop extra nutrients to support their rapid growth. Sprouts offer *twenty or thirty times more nutrients* than both the dormant seeds and the mature plants, often including some which are *only* present during sprouting. Sprouts are truly an incredible superfood.

Most nuts and seeds are more digestible after they've been soaked in lukewarm saltwater, about a teaspoon of salt per cup, for up to 24 hours. The salt helps to further deactivate the substances that interfere with digestion. Store soaked nuts and seeds in the refrigerator for 2 to 4 days, or crisp them in a dehydrator or low oven until thoroughly dry and store in a jar or sealed bag at room temperature.

These recipes also feature nuts or seeds:

SALAD DRESSINGS: *Farmgirl Ranch Dressing, Lemon Tahini Dressing, Creamy Chipotle Dressing*

SAUCES: *Creamy Dreamy Tahini Sauce, Thai Peanut or Almond Sauce, Pestos*

DIPS AND SPREADS: *Secret Hummus* (raw variation), *Mhammara Red Bell Walnut Dip, Olive-Pecan Tapenade with Pomegranate*

DESSERTS: *Cashew Dessert Cream, Lemon Cashew Cheesecake, Hazelnut Meyer Lemon Jewels, Rose-Scented Stuffed Dates, Market Fool*

BREAKFASTS: *Viking Muesli, Carrot-Tahini Butter, Cashew Hollandaise, Chia Seed Tapioca, Hippysauce Toast Spread, Macadamia Coconut Porridge, Protein Superfood Smoothie*

We've been brainwashed that food should be cheap… We have to decide that people are precious and food is precious… It won't ever be cheap to buy real food, but it can be affordable.

— ALICE WATERS,
CALIFORNIA CHEF AND FOOD ACTIVIST

HOMEGROWN SPROUTS

Yields about 4 cups

Sprouts offer an incredible array of nutrients, and they're even high in protein. Use them in salads, wraps, and sandwiches, or add them to smoothies for a nutritious boost. Growing sprouts at home costs only pennies, and is so easy!

Place in a quart-size mason jar:

1 Tbsp sprouting seeds (alfalfa, radish, broccoli, red clover, etc.)

Fill with water and cover with tight cheesecloth or a sprout screen. After 24 hours, drain the water and leave the jar tilted upside-down so water can continue to drain and air can circulate. Rinse twice per day. (Fill jar with water, swish well, and drain through the screen.) Keep it at room temperature, out of direct sunlight.

After 3–5 days, the sprouts will be ready to eat. Immerse them in a wide bowl of water and remove the hulls that float to the surface. Drain the sprouts well in a colander and store in the refrigerator.

NUT MYLK

Yields 4 cups

Use in place of dairy milk or boxed nondairy milks. I prefer to make my own, since commercial varieties still contain so many unnecessary ingredients and sugars.

Cover with lukewarm water and soak until softened (up to 24 hours):

1 cup raw seeds or nuts

1 tsp salt

Drain and rinse, then place in a blender with:

3–4 cups water, to taste

Blend very well, for up to 2 minutes. Pour through a paint strainer bag (available at hardware stores) or tight cheesecloth into a large bowl or pitcher. Squeeze to "mylk" out every creamy drop. Discard pulp or dehydrate for use as baking flour.

You can now add optional flavorings:

pinch salt (this makes a big difference in enhancing the flavor)

dash vanilla

cinnamon, cardamom, etc.

sweetener (maple, honey, dates, etc.)

Additional notes

- Hemp seed mylk is very easy to make, because it does not require straining. It also offers a lot of protein and some EFAs.
- Almond mylk has a very mild, versatile flavor.
- Brazil nut mylk is very rich and high in protein, but don't be alarmed if it has a pungency slightly reminiscent of boiled egg. It's nice in soups and smoothies with chocolate.
- Some nuts have less enzyme inhibitors than others. You can skip presoaking these, especially if they're only eaten occasionally: hemp seeds, Brazil nuts, macadamias, pistachios, pine nuts, and hazelnuts.

NUT PARM

··

Yields about 1 cup

Sprinkle on salads, pastas, polentas, risotto; anywhere you'd want
Parmesan cheese or a nutritious flavor and protein boost. I combine the
garlic and salt for a few minutes before proceeding with the recipes, to
refine the sharp garlic flavor.

Version 1

Combine and chop in food processor until finely ground:

    1 clove garlic, finely grated

    1 tsp salt

    1 cup raw Brazil nuts

Version 2

Combine and chop in food processor until finely ground:

    1 small clove garlic, finely grated

    ½ tsp salt

    1 cup almonds, toasted

    3 Tbsp nutritional yeast

    1–2 tsp *Homesteader's Honey Mustard* (DIPS AND SPREADS)

CASHEW SOUR CREAM AND CHEESES

Yields about 1 cup

Raw cashews have liberated plant-based cuisine from the mediocre tofu sauces of the past. Use this flexible, delicious recipe in place of dairy foods such as sour cream, crème fraîche, and many types of cheeses (see variations). Other nuts can make delicious cheeses too, so don't be afraid to experiment.

Basic Sour Cream:

Cover with lukewarm water and soak until softened (see notes below):

1 cup raw cashews

1 tsp salt

Drain and rinse, then place cashews in a blender with:

juice of 1 lemon

¼–½ tsp salt

Turn on the blender and slowly add:

¼–¾ cup water, to achieve desired consistency

Purée until smooth, adding water slowly to achieve the consistency you're looking for. This is the base recipe—perfect in place of sour cream.

To use in place of cheeses, you may use lemon juice, miso, and nutritional yeast, or any combination of them, or any single ingredient alone. These are the amounts I recommend:

1–3 tsp white miso, to taste

2 tsp nutritional yeast

Additional notes

- Soaked cashews only need 1–3 hours to soften, but can be left soaking up to 24 hours. If you are very short on time, just soften them with boiling water for 15 minutes.
- You may use other raw nuts for this recipe. Macadamias, pine nuts, and pistachios make particularly delicious creams and cheeses, and do not necessarily need to be soaked.

- Most cashews sold as raw are technically not, because heat is required to remove the shells. If it's important to you, you can find truly raw, hand-shelled cashews online.

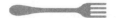

CHEESE VARIATIONS ON CASHEW SOUR CREAM

Melted Cheese

To use like a melted cheese, add just enough water to make the cream slightly pourable. You can add some red bell pepper to resemble cheddar, or chipotle powder and nutritional yeast for nacho cheese.

Cream Cheese or Chèvre

To serve like a spreadable cheese, use a minimum of water and purée the cream until it is completely smooth.

Ricotta, Queso Fresca, or Feta

To crumble on pizza like ricotta, tacos or chili like queso fresca, or on a salad in place of feta, use little or no water and use a food processor to achieve a chunky yet creamy consistency.

Herbed Feta or Chèvre

To serve like an herbed feta or chèvre, add a small grated clove of garlic, some freshly ground black pepper, 2 scallions, and 2 Tbsp mixed fresh herbs such as dill and parsley. For best flavor, treat the raw garlic as instructed in SPECIAL TECHNIQUES.

Fermented Cheese

To approximate even more closely the texture and taste of spreadable or even sliceable soft cheese, include the miso and 1 tsp unscented coconut oil. (I usually omit the lemon.) Use the least amount of water needed to purée the nuts, so the mixture isn't too wet. Transfer the cream into a cheesecloth or *nut mylk* bag, then set in a colander with a weighted plate on top. Let stand for 24 hours. It will become more tangy as it ferments.

Whipped Cream

To serve in place of whipped cream or sweet crème fraîche, see *Cashew Dessert Cream* (Desserts).

Creamy Pasta Sauce and Gravy

See *Cashew Hollandaise variations* (Breakfasts).

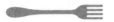

GOMASIO SALT

Yields 1 cup

This nutritious Japanese condiment is just ground sesame seeds and salt. Brown, unhulled seeds are rich in calcium, making them a better choice over hulled white seeds. Use good salt, and not too much, so you can use this flexible seasoning liberally.

Using a mortar and pestle or coffee grinder, grind together:

1 cup sesame seeds, toasted until popping and fragrant (brown or black, or a mix)

¼–1 tsp sea salt (start low and see what you like)

Store in a jar with tight lid up to 2 weeks.

Seven-Flavor Seasoning variation (Shichimi Togarashi)

- This variation makes a delicious, spicy condiment often served at Japanese restaurants. It's wonderful on noodles, rice, soups, and as a dry rub for grilling meats.

- Using a mortar and pestle or coffee grinder, grind together:
  ½ cup sesame seeds, toasted (brown or black, or a mix)
  3 Tbsp dried garlic
  2 Tbsp dried ginger or onion
  1 Tbsp Szechuan peppercorns
  3 Tbsp dulse or crushed nori
  3 Tbsp dried orange peel
  1 Tbsp crushed red pepper flakes

SUPERFOOD POWER BALLS

Yields about 12

Enjoy these easy snacks for breakfast, snack, dessert, or anytime you want a delicious healthy treat. The ingredients are powerful energy boosters and nutrient-dense superfoods. See GLOSSARY for descriptions of any that are unfamiliar to you.

Combine in food processor:

1 cup raw nuts or seeds such as walnuts, almonds, pumpkin seeds, sunflower seeds, hemp seeds, or a combination

⅓–½ cup dried dates or apricots

¼ cup goji berries

1–2 Tbsp coconut oil

1 Tbsp maca powder

1 Tbsp cacao powder

1 Tbsp raw cacao nibs

½ tsp vanilla extract

pinch salt

Process until nuts are ground and mixture is able to hold together when pressed. Form into balls using a tablespoon or hands.

Variations

- Be creative with this very flexible recipe by adding or replacing the ingredients with other superfoods or seasonings such as spirulina, honey, dried coconut flakes, tahini, almond butter, cinnamon, cardamom, and orange zest. Just balance the wet and dry ingredients so the mixture is sticky enough to hold together.
- Other dried fruits can be used, but some may require a brief soak to soften, such as figs. These should be stored in the refrigerator.

HONEY-CAYENNE PISTACHIOS

Yields 1 cup

Enjoy these on salads, as a snack, in desserts, or as substitute cashews to garnish an Indian curry.

Toast on the stovetop or in a 350° oven until barely browned, about 6–7 minutes:

1 cup raw pistachios

1 Tbsp oil

¼–½ tsp salt, to taste

While still warm, drizzle onto the seeds:

2 Tbsp honey, maple syrup, or agave syrup

½ tsp cayenne

Return to oven or stove and cook about 10 minutes more, until sticky, stirring every 2 or 3 minutes. The coating will dry as the nuts cool, so stir them occasionally while they cool or they will become more of a praline. Store in a sealed glass jar.

Variations

- Use this method to glaze other nuts, such as almonds, walnuts, pecans, or cashews.
- Use other seasonings such as curry powder, pumpkin pie spices, or citrus juice and zest.

You are what you eat.

— AMERICAN PROVERB

TUNA LOVER'S SALAD

Yields about ½ cup

Enjoy this on a sandwich or in a raw wrap of collard leaves with avocado. I like to use sweet pickles, or briefly marinate the onions in a little balsamic vinegar.

Cover with warm water and soak 7–24 hours:

¼ cup almonds

¼ tsp salt

Almonds will expand to about ⅓ cup. Drain and rinse, then place in a food processor with:

2 stalks celery, chopped

juice of 1 lemon

1 Tbsp tahini

1 Tbsp dulse

¼ tsp salt

¼ cup *Cashew Sour Cream* (NUTS AND SEEDS) (optional)

Pulse until combined but still chunky. Now add what you would like in a tuna salad. My favorite additions are:

3 Tbsp bread-and-butter pickles, chopped

¼ cup red onion, minced

1 pepperoncini, seeded and minced (optional)

chopped fresh dill and parsley

Tofu Salad variation

- This can also be made with firm tofu instead of almonds. Season crumbled tofu with some tamari, lemon, and a little nutritional yeast first, then proceed with the recipe. Add a bit of turmeric if you want it to resemble egg salad.

TAMARI-TOASTED SEEDS

I try to always have some of these around in the kitchen and at the table for garnishes or snacks.

Toast on the stovetop or in a 350° oven until barely browned and fragrant:
 raw sunflower or pumpkin seeds

While still warm, toss into the pan and stir onto the seeds:
 few dashes tamari, or shoyu

Allow the liquid to dry, briefly putting the pan back to the stove or oven if needed.

Note

- Soaked nuts or seeds can become rubbery after being toasted. If you are using soaked seeds, instead dehydrate them in a dehydrator or low oven until crisp, up to 24 hours. The slower, lower-temperature process allows them to stay crispy while preserving the live enzymes. Add the tamari at the start. Store these at room temperature in a sealed jar.

Legumes

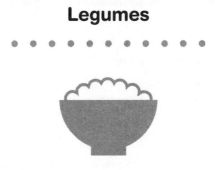

**Beans, beans, the wonderful fruit—
we've all heard the rhyme, but must it be true?**

To minimize flatulence, soak dried beans for 12 to 24 hours in enough lukewarm water to double in size. Drain and cook them in fresh water, with a stick of kombu seaweed, which can also help with digestion. If you *must* skip the long soak, try to drain and freshen the cooking water after thirty minutes of cooking. Wait to add kombu until after this step so you don't lose its vital minerals in the broth.

Salt in the soaking water will help digestibility, but salt in the *cooking* water keeps beans from absorbing water and softening properly. The exception is lentils, which do not need to be soaked—cooking these with salt will actually help them keep their shape. All others, salt them toward the end or after they've finished cooking.

One cup of dried beans, soaked overnight, is usually enough for four to six servings. Cook them slowly until they're very soft. The cooking time depends on the beans, how old they are, how long they were soaked, elevation, and other technicalities. It could be as few as twenty minutes for red lentils or as long as 2 to 3 hours for unsoaked chickpeas. Just check them and go with the flow; you can always add more water if necessary. Most beans soaked overnight won't need much more than an hour simmer.

These recipes also feature legumes:
DIPS AND SPREADS: *Secret Hummus*
SOUPS: *Coconut Masoor Dahl, White Bean Soup with Kale*
VEGETABLES: *Follow Your Heart Enchiladas*
NUTS AND SEEDS: Tofu Salad variation of *Tuna Lover's Salad*
BREAKFASTS: *Tempeh-Apple Sausage, Tempeh Sausage Hash, Tempeh Bacon*

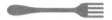

SUGGESTED AROMATICS

(To cook with dried beans)
I always add one or two sticks of kombu to add minerals, assist digestion, and reduce flatulence. It imparts rich flavor to the beans and broth. You can discard it after cooking, but I always eat it—it offers much calcium and even helps to eliminate heavy metals and radioactive particles from your body.

White Beans (Cannellini/Lima/Navy)
Bay leaf, garlic, onion, few cloves black pepper, fennel seeds, rosemary, thyme, parsley, basil, and savory.
Black/Kidney/Pinto
Bay leaf, garlic, onion, cinnamon stick, epazote (especially black beans), cumin, chili powder, and orange (with black beans).
Garbanzos (Chickpeas)
Bay leaf, garlic, onion, ginger, cardamom, cumin, black peppercorns, turmeric, coriander, fennel, cinnamon, clove, mustard seed, nutmeg, and red pepper.
Red Lentils
Same as garbanzo or white beans.

Brown or French Green Lentils

Same as white beans.

Adzuki

Ginger, garlic, onion, dried shiitakes, and Chinese five-spice blend.

Omnivorous variation

- You may want to add bones or meat to the cooking water, to add minerals and make a nourishing broth.

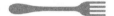

SUGGESTED ACCOMPANIMENTS

(To serve with cooked beans)

Properly cooked beans can be very satisfying served very plain, with just a little olive oil, salt, and maybe fresh herbs. Use these suggestions to pair traditional flavors with different types of beans.

WHITE BEANS, FRENCH GREEN LENTILS

Fresh Italian herbs (parsley, basil, rosemary, thyme, savory, tarragon, etc.), garlic, shallot or onion, black pepper, olive oil, balsamic or red wine vinegar, lemon, tomatoes, sautéed fennel or celery, and tomatoes.

Brown Lentils

Mushrooms, onion, garlic, fresh herbs, lemon, and olive oil.

Black/Kidney/Pinto beans

Peppers, onion, garlic, fresh cilantro, and tomatoes.

Garbanzo/Red Lentil

Indian curry spices, onion, garlic, thyme, cumin, tomato, carrot, and celery.

Adzuki

Ginger, onion, mirin, seaweed, garlic, crushed red pepper flakes, tamari, miso, toasted sesame oil, rice vinegar, and mushrooms.

FOLLOW YOUR HEART WISH BURGERS

Yields 6–10 burgers

A wish granted for meat-free burgers. Make these from leftover beans and grains, and serve them with all your favorite trimmings. Be sure to read through the entire recipe, including the notes at the end, to become familiar with the process.

Combine in a wide pan:

  1 Tbsp oil

  1 onion, diced

  1 rib celery, diced

  1 tsp salt

Cook over medium-low heat about 10 minutes, until onions begin to color. Add:

  2–3 cloves garlic, minced

  1–2 cups vegetables, chopped or grated (carrots, mushrooms, corn, peppers, etc.)

Continue to sauté until vegetables are cooked. Add:

  1–2 tsp seasoning (cumin, chili or curry powder, Italian seasoning, etc.)

  ¼ cup fresh herbs

  2–4 Tbsp water, wine, or juice

Deglaze the pan (see ESSENTIAL TECHNIQUES) and cook a few more minutes until nearly dry again.

Place in a bowl with:

  1 cup cooked beans, mashed separately

  ½–1 cup nuts or seeds, toasted (see SPECIAL TECHNIQUES) and ground

  ½–1 cup cooked grains, slightly ground in food processor

  ½–1 cup uncooked rolled oats, partially ground

Combine well with a spoon or spatula, using enough oats to make the batter sticky. Adjust salt to taste. Form patties with your hands and fry on the stovetop until browned on both sides, or coat in oil and bake in a 375° oven for 10–15 minutes each side.

ADDITIONAL WISH BURGER NOTES

- You may chill the batter for 1–2 hours prior to cooking to make a firmer patty.
- For a crunchy coating, coat the burgers in cornmeal before cooking.
- Freely exchange quantities of beans, grains, nuts or seeds, and rolled oats. The oats and cooked grains particularly help bind the batter, but a decent burger can be made without them.
- The main purpose of rolled oats is to make the batter sticky, but often the grains are enough to achieve this. You may also use flour or breadcrumbs in place of the oats.
- Any beans, grains, nuts, or seeds can work. My favorites are chickpeas, lentils, millet, short grain brown rice, walnuts, almonds, and sunflower seeds.
- See MENU PLANNING for notes about combining ingredients to create a cohesive flavor.
- The recipe for *Tempeh-Apple Sausage* (BREAKFASTS) can also be made into patties. See the variation below that recipe for notes.

Omnivorous variation

- If you eat them, cheese or eggs may be added to help bind the batter.

HOME-COOKED BLACK BEANS

Yields about 2 cups

I love black beans because they are so rich in iron and provide a lot of protein. One cup of cooked beans gives you a third of the protein you need in a day. Use these in *Smoky Chili with Butternut Squash, Follow Your Heart Enchiladas* (VEGETABLES), soups, or eat them straight up in tacos or burritos.

Soak up to 24 hours:

    1 cup black turtle beans

    3 cups warm water

    1 Tbsp salt

Drain, rinse, and place in a large pot with:

    4 cups water

    ½ yellow onion, chopped

    2 bay leaves

    1 cinnamon stick

    1 tsp cumin seeds

    1 tsp chili powder

    1–2 sticks kombu

    1 tsp epazote

Cover and bring to a boil, then reduce heat and simmer for 1–1½ hours, until soft. Drain excess cooking water and discard bay leaves. I eat the kombu separately if I don't want to use it in my recipe—it's very nutritious.

HOME-COOKED CHICKPEAS FOR HUMMUS

Yields 4 cups, or 2 cups with skins removed

Remove skins from the cooked beans for very authentic hummus. This improves their digestibility and makes the dip even creamier. The skins are very easy to pinch off, but you can skip this step if you need to. (I often do.)

Soak up to 24 hours:

1½ cups dried garbanzo beans

5 cups warm water

1 Tbsp salt

Drain, rinse, and place in a large pot with:

6 cups water

2 bay leaves

2 cloves garlic

1 Tbsp cumin seeds

1–2 sticks kombu

Bring to a boil, reduce heat and simmer up to 2 hours, until beans are well cooked. Drain water and discard bay leaves, but keep the kombu to add minerals to your hummus.

When cool enough to handle, pinch off the skins (optional).

SMOKY CHILI WITH BUTTERNUT SQUASH

Yields 4 servings

This hearty chili is very fast and easy, and you could make it even quicker by substituting canned beans and tomatoes. Make a batch of *Skillet Cornbread* (GRAINS) to serve alongside.

Prepare:

Home-Cooked Black Beans (or any combination of kidney, pinto, and black).

Save some of the cooking water to moisten the chili as needed.

Preheat oven to 425°. Combine in an oven-safe dish or pan:

1 small butternut squash, peeled and cut into 1-inch chunks

2 lb Roma tomatoes, cut into eighths

2–3 Tbsp olive oil

¾ tsp salt

½ tsp cumin

Roast for 45 minutes until soft, stirring once or twice. Set aside.

Combine in a large pot:

1 Tbsp olive oil

1 yellow onion, diced

1–3 jalapeños, seeded and diced

¼ tsp salt

Cook over medium-low heat about 10 minutes, until onions begin to color.

Add:

1 clove garlic, minced

Cook for about 3 more minutes, until garlic is fragrant.

Add:

roasted squash and tomatoes, above

2–4 chipotle chiles, seeds removed and diced

1 Tbsp chili powder

½ tsp cumin

½ tsp dried oregano, rubbed between palms

½ tsp salt

Simmer for 10 minutes, then add:

cooked beans, above

cooking water from beans, or broth or water, as needed

juice of 1 lime

Adjust salt, lime, and chiles to taste. Garnish with:

cilantro, chopped

Cashew Sour Cream (NUTS AND SEEDS)

avocado chunks

Omnivorous variations

- If you want animal protein with this vegan chili, add sautéed organic, pastured ground beef, chicken, or turkey.
- You might want to garnish this with organic sour cream or cheddar cheese.

THIS CHILI RECIPE EASILY CONVERTS INTO TWO SOUPS:

Smoky Butternut Squash Soup

Prepare the chili recipe, omitting beans and using a larger squash. Then, purée everything in batches with 4–5 cups vegetable broth (or water) in a blender and adjust seasonings to taste.

Smoky Black Bean Soup

Prepare the chili recipe with the following changes: omit the squash, double the beans, and add 1 diced celery rib and 1 sliced carrot with the garlic and jalapeños. Then, add 4–5 cups broth or water and the zest and juice of an orange. Purée half the soup in a blender, return to pot, and adjust seasonings to taste.

NEW YEAR'S BLACK-EYED PEAS

Yields 4–6 cups

Folks in the Southern US often eat these on New Year's Day to bring good luck and prosperity for the year ahead. You can also substitute a version of *Angry Sauce* (SAUCES) for the Cajun "holy trinity" (sautéed onions, green bell peppers, and celery) if you want a stovetop-free preparation. Simply omit the capers and herbs, and use green bell peppers rather than red.

Soak up to 24 hours:

 2 cups dried black-eyed peas

 5 cups warm water

 1 Tbsp salt

Drain, rinse, and place in a large pot with:

 5 cups water

 ¼ tsp peppercorns

 ½ tsp mustard seeds

 2 cloves garlic, chopped

 2 bay leaves

 1 stick kombu

Cover and bring to boil, then reduce heat and simmer for about 1 hour, until tender. Drain most of the cooking water and discard bay leaves and kombu.

Meanwhile, heat in a sauté pan:

 2 Tbsp oil

Add:

 1 yellow onion, diced

 3 ribs celery, diced

 1–2 green bell peppers, diced

 2 cloves garlic, chopped

 1 tsp salt

 ¼ tsp crushed red pepper flakes

Sauté until onions are translucent, then add:

2 lb Roma tomatoes, chopped (or one 15 oz can tomatoes)

1–2 Tbsp apple cider vinegar, to taste

Simmer until beans are cooked. Add cooked beans and some of the cooking water (as desired). Simmer for another 15 minutes and adjust salt and vinegar to taste.

Omnivorous variations

- If you want animal protein with this vegan recipe, add pieces of organic, pastured fried bacon with the tomatoes.
- You can also simmer an organic, pastured ham bone or ham hock in the water for an hour before adding and cooking the beans.

CANNELLINI BEANS WITH TARRAGON

Yields 2½ cups

Cannellinis hold their shape best of all the white beans, making them a great choice for salads. Use whichever fresh Mediterranean herbs you have in the garden or refrigerator: thyme, oregano, rosemary, marjoram, etc.

Soak up to 24 hours:

    1 cup dried cannellini beans

    3 cups warm water

    1 Tbsp salt

Drain, rinse, and place in a large pot with:

    5 cups water

    1 bay leaf

    8–10 peppercorns

    2 cloves garlic, chopped

    1–2 sticks kombu

Cover and bring to boil, then reduce heat and simmer for 1–1½ hours, until tender. Meanwhile, combine in a large bowl:

    ½ tsp salt

    1 small shallot, minced

When beans are cooked, drain and add them to this bowl with:

    2–3 Tbsp fruity olive oil, to taste

    1 tsp lemon juice

    2 tsp fresh tarragon, minced (or other herbs)

    2 Tbsp fresh Italian parsley, finely minced

Stir to combine and adjust salt to taste.

Optional additions

- Add *Rapini with Garlic and Lemon* (Vegetables), sun-dried or fresh tomatoes, roasted roots, chopped olives, baby spinach, or steamed green beans and broccoli.

Omnivorous variations

- You may want to garnish this vegan dish with freshly grated organic Parmesan cheese.

CHICKEN-FRIED TOFU

Yields 4 servings

Once considered quite healthy, tofu is now considered junk-food by many modern foodies. Decide for yourself, but this awesome recipe is for anyone who still indulges in a tofu "steak" once in a while. Serve with mashed potatoes and the Mushroom Gravy variation of *Cashew Hollandaise* (Breakfasts).

Marinate up to 1 day in the refrigerator:

1 lb firm tofu, cut into 4 servings

¼ cup tamari

1 Tbsp maple syrup

1 tsp hot sauce

Preheat oven to 350°. Transfer tofu and marinade to a baking dish and bake until pan is dry, turning once after 15 minutes.

Combine in a wide, low bowl:

½ cup flour

¼ cup cornmeal

3 Tbsp nutritional yeast

1 tsp salt

1 tsp chili powder

½ tsp black pepper

In a separate wide, low bowl, combine:

½ cup *Nut Mylk* (Nuts and Seeds)

2 Tbsp *Homesteader's Honey Mustard* (Dips and Spreads)

1 Tbsp tamari or shoyu

Dip tofu in the dry mixture, then drench in wet, and repeat once to create a thick batter coating.

Fry on both sides in a generous amount of hot oil (coconut is best). Or, brush with oil and bake at 400° until browned, turning once after about 15 minutes.

Omnivorous variations

- You can substitute regular organic milk for the *Nut Mylk*.
- You can also use this recipe to batter organic pastured chicken or meat.

INDIAN CURRY STEW
....

Yields 6 servings

No vegetarian potluck or activist event would be complete without a curried vegetable stew. This recipe highlights Indian flavors at their best, with a minimum of heavy oil. Serve it with *Coconut Jasmine Rice* (GRAINS) and perhaps offer a spicy-sweet chutney at the table.

Prepare:

Home-Cooked Chickpeas for Hummus (or use canned)

Meanwhile, heat in a soup pot:

1 Tbsp coconut oil

Add:

½ tsp cumin seeds

Fry until seeds are browned and fragrant, a few seconds. Add:

1 yellow onion, diced

1 tsp salt

Cook over medium heat until onions are translucent, about 8–10 minutes. Add:

1–2 serrano or jalapeño peppers, seeded and diced small

3 garlic cloves, minced

1 Tbsp minced or grated ginger

Cook for another 5 minutes, then add:

2 Tbsp Indian curry powder or garam masala

½ tsp each turmeric and coriander (optional if your curry powder is very fragrant)

¼ tsp crushed red pepper flakes (optional)

Cook a few minutes more, until spices are fragrant. Add:

1 cup chopped tomatoes

1 cup broth or water

2 cups red potatoes, small diced

2 cups cauliflower florets

2 cups brown mushrooms, quartered

1 tsp salt

Stir up the spices from the bottom of the pot, then cover and stew about 20 minutes until the vegetables are cooked. Stir occasionally and add water or broth if necessary to keep bottom from sticking. Add:

2 cups garbanzo beans, cooked

3 Tbsp tamarind paste, or juice of 1 lime

2 cups spinach

Adjust salt and sour to taste.

Garnish suggestions:

- Chopped cilantro
- Raw white onion, minced and marinated briefly in lime juice
- *Four-Flavor Mint Chutney* (Sauces) or Savory Chutney variation of *Dried-Fruit Compote* (Desserts)
- *Cashew Sour Cream* (Nuts and Seeds)
- *Honey-Cayenne Cashews* (Nuts and Seeds)

Omnivorous variations

- You can substitute organic butter or ghee for the coconut oil.
- You may want to garnish with organic yogurt.
- If you want to add animal protein to this vegan stew, add roasted, grilled or seared organic, pastured meats or chicken.

FABULOUS FRENCH LENTIL SALAD

Yields 2 cups

This makes a lovely picnic salad or antipasto with *Balsamic Roasted Beets* (ROASTIES). Parsley is very high in vitamin C and cleanses the blood; the finer you mince it, the more of it you can enjoy.

Place together in a medium pot:

    1 cup green French lentils, rinsed and picked through for stones

    4 cups water

    ¼ tsp salt

    2 bay leaves

    4 sprigs thyme

    1 stick kombu

Bring to a boil, then reduce to simmer for about 30 minutes, until lentils are soft. Strain and set aside. Discard bay leaves, thyme, and kombu. (I recommend eating the kombu separately for its valuable minerals.)

While lentils are cooking, combine in a large bowl and allow to marinate for at least 10 minutes:

    1 clove garlic, finely grated

    2 Tbsp balsamic vinegar

    ½ tsp salt

Add:

    cooked lentils

    ½ bunch Italian parsley (about ½ cup finely minced)

    3 Tbsp quality olive oil

    3 Tbsp kalamata olives, chopped

    zest of 1 lemon

    1 recipe Herbed Feta variation of *Cashew Sour Cream and Cheeses* (NUTS AND SEEDS) (optional)

Combine well and adjust salt to taste. Serve on a bed of:

    baby spinach or arugula

Omnivorous variations

- You can substitute organic feta cheese for the Herbed Cashew Feta.

ASIAN BRAISED TEMPEH
....

Yields 4 servings

Tempeh is from Indonesia, where it's traditionally fried in thin pieces and served as a protein-rich snack or condiment. I love the fried-food satisfaction from it, but braising tempeh uses less oil and the soft texture is a nice change. Serve this with a simple grain and steamed veggies or try it rolled up in sushi.

Preheat oven to 375°.

Combine in a small bowl:

¼ cup shoyu or tamari sauce

¾ cup apple juice

pinch crushed red pepper flakes

1½ tsp toasted sesame oil

1 large clove garlic, minced

1½-inch piece ginger, finely grated

Set aside.

Arrange in a single layer in a wide, shallow baking dish:

16 oz tempeh, thickly sliced

Pour sauce over tempeh and bake for 35 minutes. Turn each piece over at 15 minutes, adding a splash of water or apple juice if needed to avoid scorching.

Notes

- Tempeh may be marinated in the braising liquid overnight.
- Many people enjoy the texture of tempeh when it's been steamed for 10–15 minutes prior to frying or braising.

Omnivorous variations

- You can also use this recipe to braise organic pastured meats, chicken, or fish.

Grains

· · · · · · · · · · ·

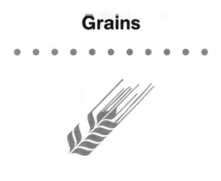

Many vegans and vegetarians who rely on whole grains are unaware that overconsumption can actually lead to mineral deficiencies. The hulls contain phytic acid, which can inhibit mineral and protein absorption if overconsumed.

Soaking, sprouting, or fermenting whole grains prior to cooking reduces this effect, and a slightly acidic soaking liquid helps break down the phytic acid even more. The simplest process is to soak grains overnight in warm water with a tablespoon of vinegar, lemon juice, whey, or yogurt per cup of grains. Drain after 12 to 24 hours, rinse, then cook as usual with a little less water than normal (see SPECIAL TECHNIQUES for more information). While this is important, it isn't necessary to be completely vigilant about soaking your grains unless your diet relies on them heavily, or if you have reason to be concerned about mineral deficiency, such as tooth decay or osteoporosis. The liquid measurements in the recipes that follow are for using unsoaked, dry grains.

Contrary to classic instruction, I don't worry too much about checking under the cover when I'm cooking grains. If they've thoroughly cooked but there's still water in the pot, just drain it off and cook them a little longer with the lid off to release the steam. If you overcook your grains, you can try to save them by laying them out on a baking sheet to evaporate some of the excess liquid. If they're undercooked, you can add more hot water and continue cooking. You'll know what to do—just pay attention to your intuition.

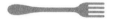

MUSHROOM RISOTTO

Yields 4–6 servings

If possible, use a combination of fresh and dried mushrooms in this recipe, such as cremini, shiitake, and porcini. Simmer dried mushrooms in the broth until they are soft enough to use.

Warm in a saucepan and keep simmering on the stove:

6 cups *Follow Your Heart Vegetable Broth* (Soups) (preferably with mushrooms)

Combine in a medium saucepan:

2 Tbsp olive oil

1 yellow onion, diced

1 stalk celery, diced

¼ tsp salt

Cook over medium-low heat about 10 minutes, until onions begin to color. Add:

3 cloves garlic, minced

1 lb mushrooms (about 6 cups), chopped

¼ tsp crushed red pepper

Sauté over medium heat about 10 minutes, until mushrooms are cooked and liquid has reduced.

Add:

1 cup Arborio rice

Stir briefly to coat with oil, then add:

⅓ cup sherry or ½ cup red or white wine

Deglaze the pan (see Essential Techniques) and simmer, stirring, until pan is nearly dry again.

Add enough to cover rice:

warm broth (about a cup)

Stir until the liquid is mostly absorbed. Repeat, adding the broth a cup or so at a time and stirring to keep the rice from sticking.

When the rice is tender (after about 35 minutes), stir in:

1 tsp salt

few twists of freshly ground pepper

¼ bunch Italian parsley, minced

Adjust salt and black pepper to taste.

Garnish each serving with:

drizzle of *Balsamic Reduction* (Desserts), or a quality balsamic vinegar

Nut Parm (Nuts and Seeds)

Omnivorous variations

- You can use organic butter in place of oil to sauté, and bone broth or milk in place of vegetable broth.
- You may want to substitute freshly grated organic Parmesan or other cheeses for the *Nut Parm*.

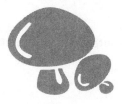

FOLLOW YOUR HEART RISOTTO

Yields 4–6 servings

Use this basic formula to make any number of risottos. Reference the additional tips in *Follow Your Heart Soup* to learn more about cooking the vegetables.

Warm in a saucepan and keep simmering on the stove:

4–6 cups vegetable broth or water

Combine in a medium saucepan:

2 Tbsp olive oil

1 onion, diced

¼ tsp salt

Cook over medium-low heat about 10 minutes, until onions begin to color. Add:

savory aromatics (garlic, celery, etc.)

assorted vegetable base (suggestions follow)

Continue to sauté until vegetables are cooked, then add:

1 cup Arborio rice

Stir to coat with oil, then add:

about ½ cup acid (wine, tomatoes, juice, etc.)

Deglaze the pan (see Essential Techniques) and simmer, stirring, until the pan is nearly dry again. Add enough warm broth to cover the rice and stir until it is mostly absorbed. Repeat, adding the broth a cup or so at a time and stirring to keep the rice from sticking. Before the rice is fully cooked, add:

fresh veggies or herbs that don't need to cook very long (peas, corn, etc.)

When the rice is tender (after about 35 minutes total), add to your liking:

about 1 tsp salt

freshly ground black pepper

fresh herbs, minced

Nut Parm (Nuts and Seeds)

Adjust salt and freshly ground black pepper to taste.

Additional Risotto-making tips

- Starchy Arborio rice is important for a true risotto. It is slightly less processed than ordinary white rice, but short-grain brown rice or pearled barley can be substituted for a whole-grain risotto.
- While water works just fine, broth will contribute much more flavor to the final dish. You may also combine other liquids with the stock, such as *Nut Mylk* (Nuts and Seeds) or juice.
- You may also cook the vegetables separately and add them after the rice is fully cooked.

Vegetable base suggestions

- Peas and Asparagus
- Roasted Butternut Squash and Sage
- Roasted Red Bell Pepper
- Sun-Dried Tomato and Red Onion
- Corn and Summer Squash

Other serving suggestions for risotto:

- Form into burger-sized croquettes and fry with a little oil. These are great with a *Pesto* (Sauces) or *Cashew Hollandaise* (Breakfasts) sauce.
- Fill hollowed-out vegetables such as squash, portobello mushrooms, or bell peppers, then roast in oven until softened. These are also nice with the creamy sauce and pestos above.

Omnivorous variations

- You can use organic butter in place of oil to sauté, and bone broth or milk in place of vegetable broth.
- You may want to substitute freshly grated organic Parmesan or other cheeses for the *Nut Parm* (Nuts and Seeds).

WILD RICE PILAF WITH CRANBERRIES AND PECANS

Yields 4–6 servings

This is an excellent recipe for the winter holidays, especially stuffed into a baked acorn squash for a vegetarian main course. The pecans will be even tastier if you coat them with oil before toasting in the oven.

Combine in a medium pot:

¾ cup brown basmati rice, rinsed

¼ cup wild rice, rinsed

2½ cups water or vegetable broth

Cover and bring to a boil, then reduce heat and simmer for 35 minutes. Remove from heat and fluff with a fork, then allow to stand, covered, for about 5 minutes. Combine with the savories below while still warm.

Meanwhile, combine in a wide pan:

1 Tbsp olive oil

1 yellow onion, diced

1 stalk celery, diced

¼ tsp salt

Cook over medium-low heat about 10 minutes, until onions begin to color. Add:

1 clove garlic, minced

¼ tsp salt

Continue to cook about 3 minutes more, until garlic is fragrant. Add:

2 cups brown mushrooms, chopped (will produce about 3 cups after they are chopped)

Sauté over medium heat about 8–10 minutes, until mushrooms are cooked. Add:

½ cup white wine

Deglaze the pan (see Essential Techniques) and simmer about 7 minutes until nearly dry again. Remove to a large mixing bowl and toss with:

warm rice (above)

⅔ cup pecans, toasted and chopped (see Special Techniques)

¼ cup cranberries

¼ cup chopped Italian parsley, and a bit of fresh sage, rosemary, savory, marjoram, or thyme

drizzle of good olive oil

Adjust salt and add freshly ground black pepper to taste.

Omnivorous variations

- You can use organic bone broth in place of water or vegetable broth, and butter in place of oil to sauté.

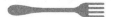

SIMPLE JAPANESE NOODLES

Yields 2–4 servings

These are a perfect accompaniment to a multi-course Japanese meal. Thanks to my sister Patricia for this simple, refined recipe.

Cook according to package directions:

8 oz udon or soba noodles

Drain and rinse with cold water. Toss with:

4 tsp toasted sesame oil

4 tsp shoyu or tamari

4 tsp rice vinegar

Garnish with:

3 Tbsp *Gomasio Salt* (Nuts and Seeds), or plain toasted sesame seeds

1 bunch scallions, sliced on the bias

Note

- Menu Planning lists other recipes that can also be served with noodles/pasta.

FOLLOW YOUR HEART PILAF

Yields 4–6 servings

Pilafs are excellent served both warm and at room temperature. Use this guide to make any variety of flavors with the ingredients you have on hand.

Prepare with water or vegetable broth:

1 cup dry grains (barley, brown rice, wild rice, etc.)

Remove from heat and fluff with a fork, then allow to stand, covered, for about 5 minutes. Combine with the savories below while still warm.

Meanwhile, combine in a medium pan:

1 Tbsp olive oil

1 onion, diced

¼ tsp salt

Cook over medium-low heat about 10 minutes, until onions begin to color. Add:

savory aromatics and assorted vegetable base, such as garlic, celery, fennel, carrot, mushroom, etc.

Continue to cook until vegetables are soft, then add:

about ½ cup wine, tomatoes, juice, broth or water

Deglaze the pan (see Essential Techniques) and simmer about 7 minutes until nearly dry again. Remove to a large mixing bowl and toss with:

warm rice (above)

⅔ cup nuts or seeds, toasted and chopped

¼ cup dried fruit

¼ cup chopped fresh herbs

drizzle of good olive oil

Adjust salt and add freshly ground black pepper to taste.

Omnivorous variations

- You can use organic bone broth in place of water or vegetable broth, and butter in place of oil to sauté.
- If you want animal protein in this vegan pilaf, add pieces of browned, organic pastured meats or chicken.

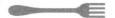

WHOLE-GRAIN SUSHI RICE

Yields 4 servings

This is a more wholesome alternative to common white sushi rice. Sweet brown rice is very sticky and sweet, and short grain rice is less of both. I usually use half and half of each type.

Combine in a medium pot:

1 cup sweet brown or short grain brown rice

2¼ cups water

1 stick kombu, about 4-inch

Cover and bring to a boil, then reduce heat and simmer for 30–45 minutes. Remove from heat and remove kombu. Fluff with a fork and allow to stand, covered, for about 10 minutes. Toss while warm with:

1½ tsp sugar (optional)

½ tsp salt

1 Tbsp + 1 tsp rice vinegar

Cool to room temperature before using for sushi.

SCATTERED SUSHI SALAD

Yields 4 servings

Invite guests to make small conical hand rolls at the table with this simple and easy way to serve a sushi meal. The variations are endless. Use the vegetables you have in whatever quantity looks good to you.

Gently combine in a large bowl:

1 recipe *Whole-Grain Sushi Rice* (previous recipe)

2 medium carrots, shredded

1 small daikon radish, shredded

3 scallions, thinly sliced

1 avocado, cubed

1 cucumber, shredded or diced small

12 large *Savory Roasted Shiitakes* (ROASTIES), sliced

pickled ginger, or *Spring Tonic Chee* (VEGETABLES)

2 Tbsp *Tamari-Toasted Seeds* or *Gomasio Salt* (NUTS AND SEEDS)

hearty sprouts, such as sunflower, mung, or pea shoots

Serve with:

nori sheets, halved

wasabi, tamari, or ume plum paste—or all three

Serve in bowls with chopsticks, or roll nori into hand-held cones and fill with this rice salad.

Note

- Pickled ginger often has artificial colors and preservatives, so read the label to be sure yours is a quality product.

QUINOA TABBOULEH

Yields 4 servings

Traditional tabbouleh is a parsley salad made with couscous, a refined semolina wheat product. I replace it with quinoa and the result is more nutritious and has a pleasing texture, too. Quinoa is one of the few plant sources of a complete protein.

Combine in a small or medium pot:

1 cup quinoa, rinsed

1½ cups water

Cover and bring to a boil, then reduce heat and simmer for 15 minutes. Remove from heat and fluff with a fork, then allow to stand, covered, for 5 minutes, fluff and set aside in a bowl.

Combine in a large bowl:

juice of 1 lemon

1 tsp salt

Add:

½ cup Italian parsley, chopped

¼ cup mint, chopped

1 cup cherry tomatoes, cut in half or quarters

1 cucumber, diced

Toss in:

cooked quinoa

generous drizzle quality olive oil

Adjust salt and lemon to taste.

COCONUT JASMINE RICE

Yields 4–6 servings

I let myself indulge in white rice very occasionally. Although it's been stripped of the nutritious exterior hull, at least the phytic acid that was in the bran isn't competing with the minerals in the rest of your meal. Moderation is the key.

Combine in a medium saucepan:

1 Tbsp coconut oil

2 cloves garlic, minced

1 Tbsp ginger, minced

1 tsp salt

Cook over medium-low heat 8–10 minutes, until onions are translucent. Add:

3 Tbsp mirin or white wine

Deglaze the pan (see Essential Techniques) and add:

1 cup jasmine rice

Stir to coat with seasonings, then add:

1 cup water

¾ cup coconut milk

Stir well, cover and bring to a boil. Reduce heat and simmer, covered, for 20 minutes. Stir once or twice during cooking to avoid burning. Remove from heat and fluff with a fork, then allow to stand, covered, for about 5 minutes.

Toss with:

grated zest from 1 lime

2 scallions, thinly sliced diagonally

Adjust salt to taste.

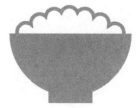

SKILLET CORNBREAD
....

Yields 12 pieces

This is a nice moist bread, and the recipe is very flexible. Try using different flours, or adjust the sweetness by exchanging maple syrup for oil. This classic skillet method makes a nice crunchy crust, but the batter can be baked in any 8 x 8-inch pan or even muffin tins.

Preheat oven to 400° and place a 9-inch cast iron skillet inside to heat up. Mix dry ingredients in a large bowl:

  1 cup cornmeal, medium or fine ground

  1 cup other flour (whole wheat, rye, pastry, etc.)

  1 Tbsp baking powder

  1 tsp salt

Whip wet ingredients in a blender for 30 seconds:

  ¾ cup oil (I prefer coconut)

  ¼ cup maple syrup

  1 cup *Nut Mylk* (NUTS AND SEEDS) or any milk

  2 Tbsp flax seeds, ground

Coat the hot skillet with oil, then stir wet ingredients into dry. Pour batter into the skillet immediately. Bake for 20–25 minutes, until a toothpick inserted into the center comes out clean. Allow to cool slightly before serving.

Variations

- Stir in the kernels from one ear of corn just before baking.
- Add up to 1 Tbsp fresh or dried herbs such as oregano, marjoram, thyme, chives, or scallions.
- Sauté 1 onion, 2 bell peppers, and 2 jalapeños with plenty of oil in the skillet, then pour batter over and bake. Check for doneness after 20 minutes.

Omnivorous variation

- You can substitute regular organic milk for the *Nut Mylk* and melted organic butter for the oil.

POLENTA FOUR WAYS

Yields 4–6 servings

Polenta is so adaptable. Serve it creamy with or without cheese, as a sweet breakfast porridge with maple syrup, in place of pasta, or even instead of rice for Latin dishes. Thanks to Alex Bury for the inspiration for the torte.

Combine in a large saucepan:

4 cups water

2 Tbsp olive oil

1 tsp salt

¼ tsp black pepper

¼ tsp crushed red pepper flakes (optional)

1 clove garlic, minced (optional)

for Italian flavors, add 1 Tbsp dried Italian herbs

for Latin flavors, add 2 tsp cumin or chili powder

Bring to a boil, then whisk in:

1 cup dried polenta

Reduce heat and simmer. Keep stirring with whisk for a minute or two, then every few minutes with a wooden spoon until the porridge is soft and no longer grainy (about 20–30 minutes).

Proceed with one of the methods that follow the variations below.

Variations

- Once cooked, you can stir in any flavorings you like: lemon zest, olives, *Nut Parm* (NUTS AND SEEDS), nutritional yeast, fresh herbs, pesto, sautéed onions and chiles, etc.
- The recipes listed to accompany pasta in MENU PLANNING are great over polenta as well.

Omnivorous variations

- You can substitute organic milk for 2 cups of the water, and use butter in place of olive oil.
- You may want to stir in ¼ cup organic sour cream and/or freshly grated Parmesan or other cheese after polenta is cooked.

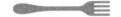

POLENTA METHODS

Creamy Polenta

The creamy polenta is ready to serve with a sauce, or add any of the flavorings listed in the variations. Pour leftovers into a pan immediately to make firm polenta, or you will need to incorporate more water when you reheat it (but the texture will suffer a little when you do this).

Firm Polenta

To make individual slices for frying or baking, pour the hot porridge into an oiled baking pan and allow to cool. Turn out and cut into squares or triangles, brush with olive oil and pan-fry or bake at 425° for about 10 minutes each side (or broil for 5 minutes each side).

Polenta Pizza

Use firm polenta in place of pizza crust by letting the porridge cool in in a wide, shallow pan. Once firm, assemble sauce and toppings. Reheat in the oven at about 425° for about 15 minutes.

Polenta Torte

Prepare 2 recipes of creamy polenta. Stir chopped spinach or a pesto into one, and a few tablespoons tomato paste into the other to color it red. Oil a deep pan, ideally springform, then pour in the green polenta. Spread a layer of Cashew Ricotta or Herbed Feta (variations of *Cashew Sour Cream*, NUTS AND SEEDS) across the top. Pour the red polenta over and refrigerate until completely firm. Slice the torte while cool and reheat individual pieces on a baking pan at 450°. Serve with *Angry Sauce* (SAUCES) and *Nut Parm* (NUTS AND SEEDS).

Desserts

Lead me not into temptation; I can find the way myself.

— RITA MAE BROWN

In my home, desserts are usually little more than a piece of perfectly ripened fruit from the farmers' market, perhaps with cream. These recipes are occasional treats, and as such many call for sugar rather than healthier substitutes. Nevertheless, I avoid conventional white and brown sugars, which are refined with chemicals and derived from genetically modified beets. Some organic sugars are refined as well. These are the various types of natural cane sugars available, which can be used interchangeably in my recipes:

Rapadura is dried sugar cane juice, dried at very low temperatures. It has a distinct molasses taste.

Sucanat is similar to Rapadura but is dried at higher temperatures.

Evaporated Cane Juice is more refined and is the closest to conventional white of all natural sugars.

Turbinado is very refined, with large crystals. I never have use for this type.

Healthful sugar substitutes include coconut sugar, honey, maple syrup, agave syrup, brown rice syrup, stevia, and date sugar. I strictly avoid unnaturally produced sugar substitutes, even including xylitol, which I am not convinced is a quality food.

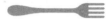

TEMBLEQUE COCONUT PUDDING

Yields 4 servings
This luscious Puerto Rican dessert is awesome by itself or cooled in a prepared pie crust.

Whisk together to completely dissolve lumps:
1 can, or 1⅔ cup full-fat coconut milk
½ cup *Nut Mylk* (NUTS AND SEEDS)
⅓ cup sugar
¼ cup non-GMO cornstarch
pinch salt
pinch nutmeg
pinch cinnamon
grated zest of half an orange
½ tsp vanilla

Combine in a small saucepan, then bring to a boil over medium heat, stirring constantly. Turn heat to low and continue to cook about 2–4 minutes, stirring well, until thickened. Pour into a bowl, a precooked pie shell, or individual glasses and refrigerate until set.

Garnish with your choice of:
orange supremes (see SPECIAL TECHNIQUES)
toasted coconut flakes
Chocolate Sauce (DESSERTS)

Omnivorous variation
- You can substitute regular organic milk for the *Nut Mylk*.

HAZELNUT MEYER LEMON JEWELS

Yields 12 cookies

This wheat- and cane sugar-free variation on Meredith McCarty's Linzer-tortes in *Sweet and Natural* is one of the best vegan cookies I've ever had. They are a sweet dream come true.

Preheat oven to 350°.

Place in a single layer in a baking dish:

1 cup raw hazelnuts

Toast until fragrant and crisped, about 10–15 minutes. Wrap in a towel to steam while they cool, then rub with towel to remove skins. Place in a food processor and chop finely.

Combine in a large bowl:

hazelnuts, above
2 cups + 2 Tbsp barley flour
¼ tsp salt
½ tsp baking powder

Combine in another bowl:

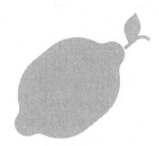

½ cup light oil
½ cup maple syrup
½ tsp vanilla
2 tsp Meyer lemon zest, chopped
1 Tbsp Meyer lemon juice

Add wet ingredients to dry and stir to make a dough. Roll into 2-inch balls and make an indentation in the middle of each for:

1 Tbsp raspberry jam

Bake jam-filled cookies on an oiled baking sheet until golden, 15–20 minutes. Allow to cool slightly before serving.

LEMON CASHEW CHEESECAKE

Yields one 9-inch cake

This raw dessert is pure decadence. Thanks to Tiziana and Matthew of Sweet Gratitude for inspiring the recipe. Exchange the liquids to adjust the flavor as you like (honey or agave syrup, lemon juice and *Nut Mylk*).

Make the crust:

Grease a 9-inch springform pan with coconut oil. Place in food processor:

  2 cups almonds, hazelnuts, or a combination

  ⅓ cup moist dates, about 10, pitted

  ¼ tsp vanilla

  ⅛ tsp salt

Process until nuts are ground and mixture is able to hold together when pressed. Lightly press this mixture evenly into bottom of pan. Set aside.

Make filling:

Place in blender:

  2½ cups cashews, soaked in water 3–24 hours and strained

  ¾ cup honey, or ½ cup agave syrup, to taste

  ¾ cup lemon juice

  1¼ cups *Nut Mylk* (NUTS AND SEEDS), to cover cashews

  2 tsp vanilla

  ¼ tsp salt

Blend for several minutes until very smooth, then add:

  scant 1 cup coconut oil, melted

Blend again to incorporate oil. Adjust sweetener and salt to taste, then pour into pan over prepared crust. Place in fridge or freezer until completely firm, up to 3 hours. Garnish with berries or thin slices of lemon.

Crust variations:

- Replace up to ½ cup nuts with cacao nibs or coconut flakes.
- Add up to ¼ cup cacao powder. Adjust dates if necessary to make the crust sticky enough.
- Try other nuts, such as pecans or pistachios.

Filling variations:

- If you prefer more or less tart, exchange measurements of lemon juice and *Nut Mylk* to taste.
- Replace liquid with equal amount of blended fruit (strawberry, mango, etc.), coffee, or other fruit juices.
- Add up to ¼ cup cacao powder.
- Add other flavorings, such as mint, cinnamon, grated ginger, or citrus zest.

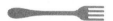

MARKET FOOL

Yields 4 servings

A fool is a traditional British dessert of whipped cream folded into seasonal fruit. Serve with *Shortbread Cookies* if you like something crunchy on the side.

Stir together:

1½ cups seasonal berries or other fruit

1 tsp lemon juice

2 tsp sugar

Allow to stand for up to 20 minutes.

Reserving some for garnish, gently fold most of the fruit mixture into:

1 recipe *Cashew Dessert Cream* (recipe follows later this chapter)

Place a small amount of fruit into separate dishes and top with fruited cream.

SHORTBREAD COOKIES

Yields 12 cookies

These simple, not-too-sweet cookies are very crumbly when they first come out of the oven, but will firm up after they cool. Serve them plain, with fruit, or drizzle them with *Chocolate Sauce* or another syrup.

Preheat oven to 350°.

Combine in a large bowl:

2½ cups flour

¾ cup sugar (add up to ¼ cup more if you like them sweeter)

¼ tsp salt

½ tsp baking powder

Stir in:

¾ cup coconut oil, melted

1 tsp vanilla

2 tsp lemon or orange zest (optional)

Form batter into 2-inch balls, place on a cookie sheet, and flatten to about ½-inch thick. Bake about 30 minutes, until golden. Remove to a plate while warm and allow to cool before serving.

Omnivorous variation

• You can substitute organic butter for the coconut oil.

> *All truth passes through three stages. First, it is ridiculed. Second, it is violently opposed. Third, it is accepted as being self-evident.*
>
> — ARTHUR SCHOPENHAUER,
> GERMAN PHILOSOPHER (1788–1860)

ROSE-SCENTED STUFFED DATES
....

These are such easy crowd-pleasers! Substitute rose water if you don't want to make your own *Rose Syrup*. Find it in Middle Eastern markets or at fine liquor stores.

Combine in a bowl:

¼ cup tahini

¼ tsp salt

¼ tsp cinnamon and/or cardamom

grated zest of 1 orange or lemon

2 Tbsp *Honey-Cayenne Pistachios* (NUTS AND SEEDS), chopped

2 Tbsp pomegranate seeds (optional)*

Place a spoonful inside each:

12 dates, pitted and halved

Arrange on a platter and drizzle with:

Rose Syrup

Garnish with unsprayed roses.

*See SPECIAL TECHNIQUES for a tip to remove pomegranate seeds easily.

Omnivorous variations

- You can add 2 Tbsp melted organic ghee to the tahini mixture.
- If you eat dairy products, try substituting the tahini with organic cream cheese or goat cheese.

CHOCOLATE SAUCE
....

Yields about 1 cup

These next four recipes are dessert sauces for fruit, cakes, and cookies. This sauce is great with a very creamy *Nut Mylk*, like coconut.

Warm in a saucepan to a low simmer:

½ cup + 2 Tbsp *Nut Mylk* (NUTS AND SEEDS)

Pour into a blender over:

1 cup dark chocolate chips

Purée until chocolate is melted and smooth.

Chocolate Ganache Frosting variation

- Reduce *Nut Mylk* to 3 Tbsp. Allow to chill in the refrigerator until it has firmed up. You can whip it with electric beaters at this point to make it lighter. The frosting is thick and firm when cool, softens into a creamy glaze at room temperature, and melts in full sun. You might also want to pour it over your cake while still wet for a smooth, thick glaze. Chill cake in refrigerator to set.

Peanut Butter Chocolate Frosting variation

- Add 2 Tbsp smooth peanut butter to the Chocolate Ganache Frosting above.

Chocolate-Dipped Fruit variation

- Use only 2 Tbsp *Nut Mylk* and dip fresh or dried fruits while sauce is still wet. Chill in refrigerator until set. Great for strawberries and dried apricots or cherries, or *Shortbread Cookies*.

Omnivorous variation

- You can substitute regular organic milk for the *Nut Mylk*.

BALSAMIC REDUCTION

Yields ¾ cup

This sweet, pungent syrup adds a deliciously sharp note to vanilla ice cream and strawberries. It's also wonderful drizzled over tomato salads, risottos, grilled vegetables, and roasted figs.

Pour into a small saucepan:

1½ cups balsamic vinegar

Simmer until reduced by half and thickened to the consistency of honey, 15–25 minutes.

Omnivorous variation

- This reduction sauce is also delicious over soft cheeses and roasted or grilled organic pastured meats, chicken, or fish.

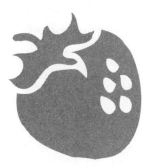

ROSE SYRUP

Yields 1 cup

This dreamy syrup adds an unexpected floral note when drizzled over fruit desserts, or added to *Cashew Dessert Cream*, lemonade, Champagne, or cocktails. Be sure the roses are unsprayed.

Combine in a small saucepan:

1 cup sugar

1 cup water

Simmer until sugar is dissolved, then add:

2 cups packed fresh rose petals (or 1 cup dried)

1 Tbsp lemon juice

Cool to room temperature, then transfer to a jar and refrigerate overnight. Strain and discard petals.

Rose Geranium variation

- Replace rose petals with 1½ cups of chopped rose geranium leaves.

Omnivorous variation

- Try drizzling *Rose Syrup* over organic whipped cream or soft cheeses.

CASHEW DESSERT CREAM

Yields about 1 cup

The recipe is a variation of savory *Cashew Sour Cream and Cheeses* (Nuts and Seeds). Use it anywhere you'd want whipped cream or a sweet crème fraîche.

Cover with warm water and soak until softened (1–3 hours, up to 24 okay):

   1 cup raw cashews

   ½ tsp salt

Drain and rinse, then place in a blender with:

   2 Tbsp sweetener of your choice

   ½ tsp vanilla

   1–2 Tbsp lemon juice, to taste (optional)

   small pinch salt

Begin to purée, slowly adding enough water to bring it to a creamy consistency (about ¼ cup, but start low—you can always add more).

Optional additions

- *Rose Syrup*, orange or lemon zest, cinnamon, brandy, or other liqueurs

HEAVENLY CHOCOLATE CAKE

Yields an 8-inch or 9-inch cake, or 12 large cupcakes

When eggs and dairy were scarce during the Great Depression, a brilliant housewife invented this inexpensive vegan recipe. Also known as Depression Cake or Wacky Cake, this moist, fluffy cake is a lot like heaven.

Preheat oven to 375°. Coat with oil, then dust with flour an 8-inch square or 9-inch round cake pan.

Combine dry ingredients in a mixing bowl:

1½ cups unbleached pastry flour, or a gluten-free blend

⅓ cup cocoa powder

1 tsp baking soda

½ tsp salt

1 cup sugar

Whip wet ingredients separately:

½ cup oil

1 cup water, coffee, or apple juice

2 tsp vanilla extract

Gently mix wet into dry ingredients. Add:

2 Tbsp apple cider vinegar

Stir well and immediately pour into prepared pan and bake for 25–35 minutes, until a toothpick poked in the center comes out clean. Allow to cool completely before removing from pan.

Frost with:

Frosting variations of *Chocolate Sauce*

Mayan Spice Cake variation

- Use balsamic for the vinegar, use coffee for water, and add 1 tsp chopped orange zest, 1 tsp cinnamon, and ¼ tsp cayenne. Top with powdered sugar.

INDONESIAN FRUIT RUJAK

Yields about 8 servings

The unexpected flavors of this spicy fruit salad will wow your guests and make them feel very worldly. It also makes a nice condiment for savory meals.

Make a peanut sauce with the following ingredients:

2 Tbsp lime juice

½ tsp salt

¼ cup peanut butter

1 Tbsp sugar, honey, or agave syrup

1–2 Thai chile peppers or up to ¼ tsp cayenne, to taste

Combine well. Toss with:

6 cups mixed fruit, such as pineapple, mango, banana, papaya, apple, watermelon, or citrus supremes (see Special Techniques)

¼ cup peanuts or almonds, toasted and chopped

2 Tbsp shallots or garlic, thinly sliced and fried crisp

Note

• Although they are not fruits, jicama and cucumber also compliment this dish nicely.

Omnivorous variation

• Indonesians traditionally add *terasi*, a strong-smelling fermented shrimp paste. You can substitute a dash of fish sauce, which you can find in Asian markets.

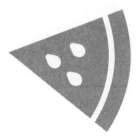

DRIED-FRUIT COMPOTE
....

Yields about 8 servings

Serve with cookies and *Cashew Dessert Cream*, as a breakfast porridge, or just enjoy it plain on a cold evening. I like it sour so I use orange juice and water, but apple juice is good if you want it sweeter.

Preheat oven to 350°.

Combine in an ovenproof dish:

   3 cups mixed dried fruit, such as apricots, cranberries, golden raisins, prunes, figs, or apples

   2 cups water, fruit juice, or a combination

   1 cinnamon stick

   1 vanilla bean, sliced lengthwise

   1 Tbsp minced ginger (optional)

   1 orange or lemon, unpeeled and sliced

Bake, stirring occasionally, until fruits are softened, about 30 minutes. Remove citrus slices and serve.

Variations

- Stovetop method: simmer for 20 minutes or until softened and liquid has reduced.
- Add toasted ground nuts, such as pistachios, pecans, hazelnuts, and walnuts.
- Add ½ cup red wine or brandy.

Savory Chutney variation

- Omit vanilla and include ginger plus half of a grated onion, ½ tsp salt, and ¼ tsp crushed red pepper. Season with lemon, lime, or balsamic vinegar before serving.

Omnivorous variation

- This recipe is also tasty with organic yogurt or vanilla ice cream.

CHOCOLATE TRUFFLES

Yields 12

These easy-to-make treats are simply a thick ganache rolled in a coating. Soften again in a double boiler if it gets too firm to work with.

Use a double boiler or set a metal bowl over a saucepan of simmering water. Combine:

¼ cup *Nut Mylk* (NUTS AND SEEDS)

1 tsp vanilla extract

1 cup chocolate chips

Stir well until chocolate is completely melted. Cool in the refrigerator up to 2 hours, until firm. Shape into balls using a spoon or tiny ice cream scoop. Coat each by rolling in a plate of:

toasted ground nuts, or

toasted coconut flakes, or

cacao powder

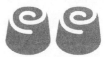

Variations

- Press a whole toasted nut into the middle of each truffle, or a *Honey-Cayenne Pistachio* (NUTS AND SEEDS).
- Add ¼ cup dried cherries or other fruit to the chocolate after it has melted.
- Replace vanilla with *Rose Syrup,* rum, brandy, or other flavorings.
- Add seasonings such as salt, cayenne pepper, grated orange zest, cinnamon, cardamom, etc.

Omnivorous variation

- You can substitute regular organic milk for the *Nut Mylk.*

PINEAPPLE RUM UPSIDE-DOWN CAKE

Yields one 9-inch cake

Like the *Heavenly Chocolate Cake*, this recipe also uses the science-fair-volcano trick of mixing baking soda and vinegar to create the volume that eggs usually provide.

Preheat oven to 350° and lightly oil a 9-inch cake pan or cast iron skillet. Reserve the juice from:

one 20 oz can unsweetened pineapple rings

Arrange pineapple rings in the bottom of the pan. Sprinkle with:

¼ cup sugar

pumpkin pie spices

grated zest of ½ lemon

Combine to make 1 cup liquid:

reserved pineapple juice, above

juice of ½ lemon

rum

Pour into a blender with:

⅓ cup coconut oil, or any oil

1 Tbsp ground flax seeds

1 Tbsp apple cider vinegar

Blend well. In another bowl, combine:

1½ cups unbleached pastry flour

1 cup sugar

1 tsp baking soda

½ tsp salt

Quickly mix wet ingredients into dry, stirring gently to dissolve lumps. Pour into oiled pan over the pineapple rings and bake for 25 to 35 minutes, or until golden and a toothpick inserted in the center comes out clean. Allow to cool. Loosen sides of cake from pan, place serving plate on top, and flip cake over onto serving plate.

Yellow Cake variation

- To make a plain yellow cake, substitute water or apple juice for the juice and rum. Proceed with recipe, with or without fruit at bottom of pan.

Breakfasts

· · · · · · · · · · ·

Some of these recipes are very simple, such as the *Viking Muesli* or *Chia Seed Tapioca*. Prepare these in the evening to be ready to eat in the morning before work or school. Others, such as the *Tempeh Sausage Hash* and the *Summer Benedict*, are for brunch feasts when you have more time. Whichever way you prepare your breakfast, I hope you will always begin your days nourished, inspired, grateful, and at ease.

These recipes are also great for breakfast:

ROASTIES: *Roasted Root Medley, Savory Roasted Shiitakes, Creamy Tahini-Coated Roasties*

VEGETABLES: *Rapini with Garlic and Lemon*

NUTS AND SEEDS: *Superfood Power Balls*

LEGUMES: *Follow Your Heart Wish Burgers*

GRAINS: *Risotto* formed into patties, *Polenta* (especially creamy as a porridge), *Skillet Cornbread, Coconut Jasmine Rice*

DESSERTS: *Market Fool, Dried-Fruit Compote, Indonesian Fruit Rujak*

SUMMER BENEDICT
....

Yields 6 servings

You will need to multitask to get this meal on the table hot, or you can prepare everything ahead and simply reheat when you're ready to serve. This recipe is also great served at room temperature, so no worries!

Prepare:

    1 recipe *Firm Polenta* (GRAINS)

    2 red bell peppers, roasted (see SPECIAL TECHNIQUES) and cut into 6 pieces total

    1 large bunch spinach, sautéed or lightly steamed

Preheat oven to 425°.

Toss each with olive oil and salt, and place in baking dishes:

    6 portobello mushroom caps, whole, remove stem and gills with a spoon

    2 large tomatoes, thickly sliced

    2 red onions, thickly sliced

Roast for about 30 minutes, until cooked.

Cut polenta into 6 pieces and brush with olive oil. Place in an oven-safe dish and reheat for 10–15 minutes. On each plate, stack:

    1 roasted portobello mushroom cap

    1 slice polenta

    1 slab roasted red bell pepper

    cooked spinach

    1 slice roasted tomato

    1 slice roasted red onion

Top with:

    Cashew Hollandaise Sauce (recipe follows on page after next)

Serve immediately.

Variations

- Add or substitute summer squash, eggplant, or baked tofu.
- Add or substitute a *Pesto* (SAUCES) for the *Hollandaise*.

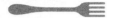

HIPPYSAUCE TOAST SPREAD

This incredible combination is inspired by a favorite on the menu at a cool, short-lived café by the same name in West Oakland. The spices are anti-inflammatory and assist digestion. This recipe also makes a fantastic dessert snack.

Combine well:

1 cup almond or peanut butter

1¼ cups honey or maple syrup

1 Tbsp salt

1 Tbsp cardamom

1 Tbsp turmeric

1½ Tbsp cinnamon

¼–½ tsp cayenne

⅓ cup coconut oil

Spread liberally on toast, apples, or hearty sourdough bread fried in coconut oil.

Omnivorous variation

- This is also delicious with organic butter or ghee in place of the coconut oil.

CASHEW HOLLANDAISE SAUCE

Yields 6 servings

I created this rich sauce as a dairy-free alternative to hollandaise sauce, but you can easily alter it to make a pasta sauce or gravy (see variations). You can use other nuts as well; try walnuts, macadamias, or pistachios.

Cover with lukewarm water and soak until softened (1–3 hours, up to 24 okay):

1 cup cashews

¼ tsp salt

Drain and rinse, then place cashews in a blender with:

grated zest and juice of 1 lemon

½ tsp salt

1 clove garlic, finely grated

1 Tbsp nutritional yeast

dash cayenne pepper

1¼ cups *Follow your Heart Vegetable Broth* (Soups) (ideally with mushrooms)

Purée until creamy, using more broth if necessary to achieve a creamy consistency. Adjust seasonings to taste.

Creamy Pasta Sauce variation

- Add fresh mixed herbs and ¼ tsp freshly ground black pepper. Try it over fettuccini with *Savory Roasted Shiitakes* and *Tempeh-Apple Sausage* or *Tempeh Bacon*.

Mushroom Gravy variation

- Omit lemon, add ½ lb *Savory Roasted Shiitakes* (Roasties) and up to ½ tsp freshly ground black pepper.

MACADAMIA COCONUT PORRIDGE

These next three recipes for satisfying breakfast cereals are very simple to prepare. This one, a classic from Café Gratitude, is also delicious with pecans and strawberries (but always include an apple for texture).

Place in blender:

1 large apple, cored and roughly chopped

water and flesh of 1 young coconut

½ cup macadamia nuts

½ tsp vanilla

dash cinnamon

pinch salt

Pulse to a chunky consistency (or smooth, if you prefer). Don't forget the salt, which will enhance the flavor even though this is a sweet porridge.

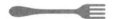

CHIA SEED TAPIOCA

Yields 1 serving

This delicate, silky pudding makes a quick and simple breakfast or dessert. I also appreciate it very plain, with just the seeds and fresh *Nut Mylk*. Chia seeds are one of the richest plant sources of omega-3 oils.

Combine well and allow to soak at least 30 minutes, up to overnight in the refrigerator:

2 Tbsp chia seeds

6 oz *Nut Mylk* (Nuts and Seeds) or coconut milk

dash of vanilla extract

dash of cinnamon

small pinch salt

Stir well and serve with:

swirl of honey or maple syrup

fresh berries or other seasonal fruit

VIKING MUESLI

Thanks to my friend Simran Skie's Norwegian roots for the inspiration! I always keep a big batch on hand in the pantry. Soaking muesli is a traditional preparation; read the introductions to NUTS AND SEEDS and GRAINS to learn about why it's important.

Combine the dry mix:

4 cups rolled grains: oats, rye, triticale, etc.

4 cups any combination of dried fruit and raw seeds or nuts: raisins, cranberries, currants, date pieces, cashews, sunflower seeds, sesame seeds, almonds, walnuts, candied ginger, etc.

FOR 1–2 SERVINGS

Combine in a large mason jar or bowl:

1 cup dry mix, above

1 cup *Nut Mylk* (NUTS AND SEEDS)

1 Tbsp lemon juice

pinch salt

Soak overnight. In the morning, add:

1 cup grated apple, or other fresh fruit

¼ tsp cinnamon (optional)

dash vanilla extract (optional)

additional *Nut Mylk* or the water and flesh of a young coconut (optional)

Variations

- To make a warm cereal, add ½–1 cup more water or *Nut Mylk* after soaking and simmer for 3–5 minutes.

Omnivorous variation

- Muesli is traditionally soaked with yogurt in place of *Nut Mylk* and lemon. If you do this, add a little water or regular organic milk to the soak if needed to moisten it enough that the dry mix can swish around a little when first added. I like to add more organic yogurt or milk in the morning, in place of the *Nut Mylk* or young coconut.

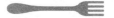

CARROT-TAHINI BUTTER

Yields 1 cup

This was always on our breakfast buffet at the Macrobiotic Café in Oakland, sometimes using beets or parsnips instead of carrots. The vegetables may also be steamed, which can retain more of their nutrients.

Bring to a boil in a medium pot:
   4 cups water
   1 tsp salt

Add:
   2 cups carrots, chopped (about 4)

Cook until very soft, 10–15 minutes. Strain and reserve some of the water.

Combine in a food processor:
   cooked carrots
   1–2 Tbsp tahini, to taste
   ¼–½ tsp salt, shoyu, or tamari, to taste

Process until smooth, adding about 3–4 tablespoons water from cooking carrots as needed to achieve a creamy consistency.

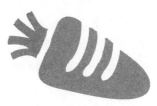

TEMPEH-APPLE SAUSAGE

Yields about 1½ cups

This is also awesome as a pizza topping or over pasta with marinara or Creamy Pasta Sauce (variation of *Cashew Hollandaise*). I like to steam the tempeh for 10 minutes first, but it's great even if you skip that step.

Heat in a wide skillet over medium heat:

3 Tbsp coconut oil

When oil is hot, add:

8 oz tempeh, steamed and cut into about ¼-inch cubes or crumbled

Fry until browned and barely crispy. Adjust the heat as necessary so as not to smoke the oil. Just at the end, add:

few splashes tamari or shoyu

Immediately turn out onto a paper towel. Set aside.

Combine in a skillet over medium heat:

1 Tbsp olive oil

½ yellow onion, diced

½ stalk celery, diced small

⅛ tsp crushed red pepper

½ tsp salt

Cook about 10 minutes, until onions begin to color. Add:

3 cloves garlic, minced

½ apple, peeled and diced small

½ tsp dried sage

1 Tbsp fennel seeds, toasted and ground

½ tsp chili powder

few twists freshly ground black pepper

Cook for 3–4 more minutes, until garlic is fragrant. Add:

3 Tbsp apple juice

Deglaze pan (see ESSENTIAL TECHNIQUES) and simmer for just a few minutes, until liquid reduces but pan is not completely dry. Add:

    fried tempeh, above

Stir well and adjust salt to taste.

- To make patties, crumble completed recipe with a few tablespoons of flour and combine well. Press into ¼-inch thick patties and fry or bake 5–10 minutes, until browned.

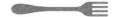

TEMPEH SAUSAGE HASH

Yields 6 servings

Addictive! Use red or yellow potatoes, or substitute up to 1 cup sweet potatoes. I'd serve this with a side of *Rapini with Garlic and Lemon* (VEGETABLES).

Combine in a large skillet over medium heat:

    1 Tbsp olive oil

    ½ yellow onion, diced

    1½ lb potatoes, cut into small cubes (about 3 cups)

    ½ tsp salt

Cover and cook over medium heat until potatoes begin to soften, stirring occasionally. Add:

    ¼ cup apple juice

    ½ tsp tamari

    pinch crushed red pepper

    ½ tsp chili powder

Use the liquid to deglaze pan (see ESSENTIAL TECHNIQUES) then add:

    2 cups chopped mushrooms (about 1 cup whole)

    Sauté until vegetables are thoroughly cooked. Stir in:

    1 recipe *Tempeh-Apple Sausage*

Adjust salt and freshly ground black pepper to taste.

TEMPEH BACON

Yields 3–4 servings

This is much simpler than the *Tempeh-Apple Sausage*, and just as tasty. You can steam the tempeh for 10 minutes first to make it more moist, but it's great either way. Use a quality oil, because the tempeh will absorb a good amount of it.

Heat in a wide skillet over medium-high heat:

2 Tbsp coconut oil

When oil is hot, add:

8 oz tempeh, thinly sliced

Fry until golden brown and barely crisped on both sides. Sprinkle evenly over tempeh in pan:

1 Tbsp apple cider vinegar

2 Tbsp tamari

2 tsp maple syrup

few dashes of hot sauce

1 Tbsp nutritional yeast

Stir and cook just long enough to incorporate flavors and absorb most of the liquid. Finish with a light sprinkle of:

smoked salt (optional)

> *There is no fundamental difference between man and animals in their ability to feel pleasure and pain, happiness, and misery.*
>
> — CHARLES DARWIN

PROTEIN SUPERFOOD SMOOTHIE

Yields 1 serving

Commercial protein powders usually contain synthetic ingredients, but the hemp seeds, almond butter, and spirulina in this smoothie offer about 25 grams of whole food protein. This recipe also provides antioxidants, essential fatty acids, chlorophyll, vitamins, minerals, electrolytes, and mood-elevating energy. A perfect meal on the go.

Combine in a blender to make the *Nut Mylk*:

3 Tbsp hemp seeds

½ cup young coconut water, fruit juice, or plain water

Blend well, then add:

1 Tbsp almond butter

1 frozen banana

¼ cup frozen berries

1–3 tsp spirulina, or a handful of greens

2 Tbsp cacao powder

1 Tbsp maca powder

1 Tbsp coconut or flax oil

¼ tsp vanilla

pinch salt

pinch cinnamon

¼ cup young coconut flesh (optional)

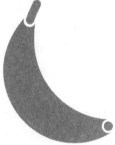

Blend again until smooth.

Omnivorous variation

- If you want dairy products in this smoothie, substitute organic milk for the young coconut water and yogurt for the young coconut flesh. Use flax oil rather than coconut.

FOLLOW YOUR HEART MUFFINS

Yields about 12 muffins

Use this basic recipe to make any variety of dairy-free muffins. I soak the flour with the water and lemon overnight to reduce the phytic acid (see introduction to GRAINS). If you do this, just stir in the rest of the ingredients when you're ready to bake.

Preheat oven to 350°.

Combine dry ingredients:

1½ cups unbleached pastry flour, or a gluten-free blend

1 tsp baking soda

½ tsp baking powder

¼ tsp salt

Combine wet ingredients:

1 cup water

½ cup liquid sweetener (honey, maple syrup, etc.)

3 Tbsp oil

1 tsp vanilla extract

2 Tbsp ground flax seeds

1 Tbsp lemon juice

Stir wet ingredients into dry and immediately pour into oiled muffin tins. Bake for 15–20 minutes, until a toothpick inserted in the middle comes out clean.

Optional additions:

½ cup dried fruit

½ cup chopped nuts or seeds

1 Tbsp poppy or sesame seeds

1 tsp citrus zest

1 Tbsp grated fresh ginger

1 Tbsp fresh herbs

½ cup sautéed savories, such as onions, peppers, corn, etc.

Rose Syrup (DESSERTS) drizzled over finished muffins

Acknowledgments

First and foremost, I am indebted to the women of Angela Farmer's annual yoga retreat in Northern California for calling forth the original version of this book. The recipes were inspired by my menu plans for this potent group, and I am so grateful to have had their support and encouragement to create this offering.

Thanks to Brenda Knight and all the helpful, encouraging staff at Viva Editions for inviting me to have it published, and thanks also to Berkeley's Ecology Center store for making the connection for us. The first edition of this book was self-published as *Piece of My Heart*, and *Vegan*ish wouldn't exist without the generous friends who made that first effort possible. Thank you, dears Malcom Scott, Jon Marro, Joshua Bates, and Ali and Mahrou Mirabdal.

My deep gratitude goes to my heart-sister Patricia Lawrence, my daughter's godmother Patty, for her reluctant midwifery of yet another project. My life wouldn't look the same without her devoted help. I love you, girlfriend. Huge thanks also to my mama, Diane Chénier, whose unconditional love and generous support stretches me into receiving what I need even when it's uncomfortable to do so. And sweet thanks to my patient daughter, Clara Rose, for her continued flexibility and joyfulness through this process.

I am grateful to all my friends and family who tested and tasted the recipes, and patiently listened to me go on and on about how to put this book together. Special thanks to little James Bird for his especially enthusiastic feedback, and to his mother, Stephanie, for sharing the encouraging stories of her dedicated recipe testing. My brother Erin, his wife Nicole, and friends Orchid, Malcom, Teri, Jonathan, Patricia, Hoss, Sadie, and Joshua also laboriously tested recipes for me. Thanks to Patricia, Jade, Tizi, Matthew, Terces, Orchid, Simran, and Meredith for letting me use your wonderful recipes.

Thanks to Hillary Curtis for urging me to value myself and be worthy of the abundance I receive, and to Matty and Terces Engelhart, owners of Café Gratitude, for introducing me to the concept that I am the source of my experience regardless of my circumstances. Thanks also to all the friends and family who have supported me when the going gets rough. You know who you are, and I do too. Thanks.

My gratitude to the chefs who have taught and inspired me: Alex Bury, Chandra Gilbert, Patricia Lawrence, Jade Mariconi, Terces Engelhart, Meredith McCarty, Eric Tucker, Alice Waters, and Deborah Madison, to name a few.

Thank you to John Robbins, for his teachings and open-minded devotion to universal well-being, and for his book *Diet for a New America*, which changed my life at sixteen years old. Thanks also to Ramiel Nagel, for changing my life again twenty years later with his book *Cure Tooth Decay*. I'm disturbed but grateful (see INTRODUCTION).

And of course, dear reader, I am grateful to you: for being curious and open to the possibility of cooking vegan*ish*, whatever your diet may be; for being willing to explore balance; and for loving yourself enough to eat well. You inspire me.

Finally, I give thanks to Mama Nature for guiding me and teaching me just about everything I know. May I always be open to the transformations she offers.

Sources of Additional Information

Just a few suggestions, and by no means a comprehensive list of the vast collection of excellent resources for cooking and healthy living.

COOKBOOKS

The Art of Fermentation and *Wild Fermentation*, by Sandor Katz, are the
go-to books for krauts and ferments.

The Art of Simple Food, by Alice Waters, is a lovely, approachable book
with easy instructions and great suggestions for eating well.

Complete Vegetarian Kitchen, by Lorna Sass, has very helpful grain and
bean cooking reference charts and good recipes for healthy cooking.

Culinary Artistry, by Andrew Dornenburg and Karen Page, is an incredible reference book for dedicated foodies. It provides endless charts of
flavors and pairings, as well as discussions of flavor and menu composition.

The Essential Vegetarian Cookbook, by Diana Shaw, is a fantastic textbook for vegetarian cooking.

I Am Grateful, by Terces Engelhart and Orchid, is a book of inspired raw
cuisine from the acclaimed restaurant Café Gratitude, where I cooked
for four years.

Healing with Whole Foods, by Paul Pitchford, is a valuable resource about nutrition, general health, and Chinese medicine, with recipes.

The Millennium Cookbook, by Eric Tucker, is a vegan cookbook with easy-to-follow advanced techniques and unique recipes, including excellent desserts by Sascha Weiss.

Nourishing Traditions, by Sally Fallon, is an extreme but interesting book that revives traditional cooking methods, focusing heavily on animal-based foods. Great reference for making bone broths.

Rainbow Green Live-Food Cuisine, by Gabriel Cousens, MD, describes how to heal chronic disease with living foods.

Sweet Gratitude, by Tiziana Alipo Tamborra and Matthew Rogers, is an innovative raw desserts cookbook, also from Café Gratitude.

Sweet and Natural, by Meredith McCarty, is my favorite resource for naturally sweetened vegan desserts.

Vegetarian Cooking for Everyone, by Deborah Madison, is an incredible guide for all levels with very refined, simple recipes.

FILMS

Some interesting, relevant, and occasionally shocking movies about human health, animal suffering, and environmental destruction:

American Meat: A pro-farmer look at chicken, hog, and cattle production in America, featuring Joel Salatin of Virginia's revolutionary Polyface Farms (2013).

Cafeteria Man: An entertaining documentary about a chef's effort to over-haul Baltimore school lunches with locally grown, freshly prepared foods (2011).

Earthlings: A graphic movie about humanity's use of animals as pets, food, clothing, entertainment, and for scientific research (2005).

Fast Food Nation: The dark side of the All-American Meal (2001).

Forks Over Knives: The plant-based way to health (2011).

Food Inc.: An unflattering look inside America's corporate-controlled food industry (2008).

Food Matters: A documentary about the causes and natural treatments of modern illnesses (2009).

The Future Of Food: An investigation into genetically engineered foods (2004).

Genetic Roulette: The Gamble Of Our Lives: An exposé about GMOs by leading authority Jeffrey Smith (2007). Book also available.

King Corn: A documentary showing how corn industrialization has all but eliminated the image of the family farm (2007).

May I Be Frank: An inspiring independent film following the 42-day transformation of an obese, sick, depressed, addicted man who is coached to wellness by three young men from Café Gratitude (2010).

Meet Your Meat: A graphic 12-minute documentary of factory farm conditions (2003). Watch online for free at www.meat.org.

Supersize Me: A documentary following a man who ate only McDonald's food for 30 days (2004).

WEBSITES ABOUT ANIMAL AGRICULTURE

www.egglabels.com
Humane Society of the United States guide to egg labels and animal welfare

www.meatanddairylabels.com
Humane Society of the United States guide to meat and dairy labels and animal welfare

www.peacefulprairie.org/freerange1.html
A moving account of a visit to a "free-range" farm, by a woman who runs a farm animal sanctuary

www.eatwild.com and www.localharvest.org
Sources for sustainably grown animal foods

www.animalwelfareapproved.org
Offers a free smartphone app that deciphers the terms used on food labels

WEBSITE RESOURCES FOR HEALTHY LIVING

www.cornucopia.org/who-owns-organic/

A link to a chart that shows how many of the natural and organic brands are owned by mainstream junk-food corporations, many of whom financially support the blocking of GMO labeling initiatives and other unethical endeavors. This is great information for those who care to use their money to "vote" for who controls our food system and public access to important information.

www.curetoothdecay.com

This is the book I used to heal my daughter's severe Early Childhood Tooth Decay (ECTD). The website is very generous with helpful information.

www.ecologycenter.org/factsheets/

A website for the Ecology Center in Berkeley, California. I especially appreciate their fact sheet about plastics.

www.ewg.org

The Environmental Working Group publishes The Dirty Dozen list of most-pesticide-laden produce, and is an excellent resource for learning about toxics in cosmetics, sunscreens, cellphones, and other consumer products.

www.feelgreatchocolate.com

From Coracao Confections, a gourmet raw chocolate company, with excellent information about the health benefits of cacao and other superfoods.

www.gapsdiet.com

Gut and Psychology Syndrome: Using diet to successfully treat autism, learning disabilities, neurological disorders, psychiatric disorders, immune disorders, and digestive problems.

www.greenfootsteps.com/cleaning-with-salt.html
In the chapter ABOUT SALT, I suggested that conventional refined table salt should be used for cleaning rather than cooking. This website describes how to do so.

www.johnrobbins.info and www.foodrevolution.org
Resources and inspiration from author and activist John Robbins and his son Ocean. The food revolution site has a great discussion about grass-fed beef from 2012.

www.localharvest.org
Find farmers' markets, family farms, and other sources of sustainably grown food in your area, or order online things you can't find locally.

www.kitchenstewardship.com/seriescarnivals/soaking-grains-an-exploration/
A very helpful discussion about reducing phytic acid in grains.

www.mercola.com
Dr. Joseph Mercola's website of cutting-edge, often unconventional, natural health advice.

www.nourishingherbalinfusions.com
Learn to brew herbal infusions to supplement important nutrients in your diet.

www.responsibletechnology.org
The most comprehensive online source of GMO health risk information and action alerts.

www.veganhealth.org
An interesting website by dietician Jack Norris, offering his solutions to the dilemma of reconciling the nutritional difficulties of a vegan diet with the commitment to reduce animal suffering. Offers important discussions about factors such as vitamin B12, calcium, and essential fats.

Glossary

**Some of the following ingredients may be unfamiliar,
and what I share about others may surprise you.**

Arame is a mild sea vegetable rich in minerals and vitamins. Usually sold in tiny strands, it can be reconstituted and added to soups, sautéed vegetables, stews, or salads.

Broccoli rabe, or **rapini,** is a brassica green-leaf vegetable related to turnips. The name refers to the broccoli-like buds that grow between the leaves. The flavor is nutty and slightly bitter.

Burdock, or **Gobo,** is a slender, elongated root vegetable with a strong, earthy flavor. Use it like a carrot. It is very nourishing, purifying, and balancing, particularly for the blood, liver, and kidneys. I always include the peel, which seems very dirty but is cleansed sufficiently by a gentle scrubbing.

Cacao powder, bits, or nibs are simply chocolate beans, same as cocoa. Natural cacao manufacturers often use this spelling to differentiate pure cacao from mainstream cocoa, which may contain corn syrup solids,

GMO sugar, chemical preservatives, and other low-quality ingredients. Natural cacao offers powerful antioxidants and boosts serotonin and endorphins, enhancing mood, energy levels, and overall well-being. See Sources of Additional Information for websites to learn more about the health benefits of moderate natural chocolate consumption.

Capers are the pickled buds of a Mediterranean flower related to nasturtiums, usually sold in jars. Their flavor is sour and salty, reminiscent of olives. I often rinse them prior to using.

Chipotle chiles are smoked red jalapeños. The flavor is smoky, sweet, and spicy. Purchase dried, powdered, or in cans with adobo sauce. Use the sauce in place of the chile peppers themselves if you prefer it less spicy. I usually remove the seeds, because they are too spicy for most palates.

Coconut oil is an antifungal, antiviral, and antibacterial cooking oil, and is excellent for skin care as well. The oil hardens at lower temperatures and can be softened by gently warming it. Depending on the brand, coconut butter can refer to either the hardened oil or to a blend of oil and coconut flesh. Early studies confused many people about its healthfulness, because they used *hydrogenated* coconut oil. The type of saturated fat in pure coconut oil is different from other types of saturated fats, and is actually quite beneficial.

Young coconut, usually imported from Thailand, is a green coconut, usually sold with the outer shell trimmed off and wrapped in plastic. These are white with a flat bottom and pointy top. See Essential Techniques for instructions to open them. The water is slightly sweet and very nutritious, high in electrolytes, potassium, minerals, and antioxidants. The white flesh is usually of a jelly consistency, perfect for smoothies and delicious for snacking. Choose coconuts that are mostly clean white, especially across the bottom. Pink or black shades often indicate spoilage.

Cremini mushrooms are small brown mushrooms with a better flavor and texture than common white button mushrooms.

Goji berries are small dried red berries from Asia. They are tart and sweet, and high in antioxidants, which help prevent cancer and boost the immune system. Snack on them like raisins, or add to salads, soups, teas, rice, desserts, muffins, and muesli.

Hijiki is a sea vegetable very rich in calcium, iron, protein, and other important nutrients. Soak one teaspoon of dry hijiki per serving for ten minutes to rehydrate into small spaghetti-like pieces (it quadruples in size). I often use this as a nutrition-boosting condiment, sometimes seasoned with a little shoyu or toasted sesame oil.

Kombu, or **kelp,** is a nutrient-rich sea vegetable that can increase the digestibility of beans and grains. It also improves the flavor and nutritional value of soups. It eliminates heavy metals and radioactive particles from the body. I add one or two 4-inch pieces to every pot of beans or grains I cook.

Maca is a root from South America, usually sold as a powder. It increases stamina, helps with fatigue, and boosts sexual functioning (libido, fertility, etc.). Its malty, slightly nutty flavor is delicious in smoothies.

Mirin is a sweet Japanese cooking wine made from fermented rice. Read the label to make sure it has not been sweetened with corn syrup.

Miso is a fermented soy bean paste that can also be made from grains or other beans. Usually salty, some varieties can also be slightly sweet. White miso and natto miso are more mild; red and brown are more pungent. Add it to soups, sauces, dips, marinades, or other dishes after cooking to preserve the heat-sensitive beneficial live cultures.

Nori is a sea vegetable sold in thin sheets and used to wrap sushi. It's rich in vitamin C and offers plenty of minerals and protein. It also makes a crunchy snack right out of the package.

Nutritional yeast is a yellow powder used as a flavor-enhancing supplement, often to resemble the flavor of cheese. It can convert to a potential excitotoxin (MSG) when processed with high heat. A light yellow color indicates lower temperature processing—one brand I can recommend is Frontier. I use nutritional yeast sparingly, but it can easily be omitted from any of my recipes. It is not the same as brewer's yeast. Nonorganic brands are likely cultured on genetically modified sugars.

Parsley is a very nutritious herb, high in vitamins, minerals, and antioxidants. I prefer flat-leaf Italian parsley over the more bitter common curly type, because it is more flavorful and more closely resembles the wild variety. It grows easily in a backyard garden or pot.

Pepita is a Spanish culinary term for a toasted pumpkin seed. Pepitas are a crunchy, iron-rich garnish for any meal.

Pistou is a cold sauce usually made of minced garlic, oil, salt, and fresh herbs. It can be served as a soup garnish, with pasta, or as a dip for bread. It may be made by omitting nuts from my pesto recipes.

Portobello mushrooms are mature cremini mushrooms, great for roasting or grilling whole. The large size and meaty taste and texture makes them good substitutes for burgers.

Shiitake mushrooms are medicinal edible mushrooms that support the immune system and help prevent disease. The dried mushrooms may have even more nutritional value. Reconstitute these by simmering in water for 20 minutes. Retain the flavorful water to use in soups or for cooking grains.

Shoyu, soy sauce, and **tamari** are terms often used interchangeably, but they do have traditional meanings that are becoming more standardized in labeling. *Tamari* is a Chinese sauce made of soybeans and little or no wheat. *Shoyu* is a Japanese sauce made of equal parts soybeans and wheat, usually a little sweeter than tamari. Traditionally, both require many months of fermentation. Ordinary mass-produced *soy sauce,* which is chemically extracted in a matter of days, usually contains unhealthy additives such as corn syrup, artificial colors, and preservatives. Always read the ingredients and look for the term *naturally fermented* on the label. I do not use the liquid soy sauce substitute sold in health food stores because it is rumored to be chemically produced in a similar way to ordinary soy sauce.

Smoked paprika is a dried Spanish seasoning that is smoky, slightly bitter-sweet, and mildly spicy.

Smoked salt is a very special finishing salt with a strong smoky flavor, made in a wood smoker. It particularly complements mushrooms and tomatoes. Avoid smoke *flavored* salt; it is unnaturally flavored.

Stevia is a plant that is three hundred times sweeter than sugar. Just a couple drops of stevia extract can replace sugar in a recipe. Try different brands until you find one you like; some products can leave a noticeable aftertaste that many people find unpleasant.

Tahini is a ground sesame seed paste traditionally used in Asian, Middle Eastern, and eastern Mediterranean foods. It is available raw or toasted, which has a deeper, nuttier flavor. Unhulled sesame seeds are very high in calcium, but a tahini paste made from whole seeds can be difficult to find unless ordered on the internet.

Tamarind is a very sour, somewhat sweet fruit from a pod, used in Asian, Indian, African, and Latin cooking. The paste is sold by the block or in a jar. If you buy it in blocks, soften a chunk for your recipe in a little hot water and push the paste through a sieve to separate from the large seeds.

Tempeh is a block of cooked, fermented soy beans that may also contain grains or other beans. The enzymes from fermentation make it the most digestible form of soy. Brown spots are fine, but a pink color indicates spoilage. Tempeh is from Indonesia, where it's traditionally fried in thin pieces and served as a protein-rich snack or condiment. You may steam or marinate (or both!) prior to frying, braising, or cooking any other way.

Ume, or **umeboshi paste,** is a tangy, salty Japanese condiment made of pickled umeboshi plums. A digestive aid, it can be used in sushi, dips, dressings, or sauces, or spread on steamed broccoli or corn on the cob in place of salt and butter.

Wakame, or **alaria,** is a delicate, mild-tasting sea vegetable that's rich in minerals and vitamins. Break it into smaller pieces before adding to soups or reconstituting in water for salads.

Wasabi is a spicy, mustardy paste usually served as a condiment with sushi. Traditionally made from a rare Japanese horseradish, most packaged varieties are regular horseradish with mustard and artificial green coloring. Read the label to be sure you are purchasing a natural product without artificial colors.

Zest is the outermost skin of a citrus fruit, used for a bright note of flavor. Always use organic fruit, and avoid the bitter, inner white layer when removing zest.

Index of Recipes

Helpful Culinary Conversions

3 teaspoons = 1 Tablespoon

4 Tablespoons = ¼ cup

⅓ cup = ¼ cup + 1 Tbsp + 1 tsp

1 cup = 16 Tbsp, or 8 fluid ounces

1 pint = 2 cups, or 16 fluid ounces

1 quart = 4 cups, or 32 fluid ounces

1 liter = 34 fluid ounces, or 1 quart + ¼ cup

1 gallon = 4 quarts, or 128 fluid ounces

FOR TRUE ACCURACY

- Dry ingredients should be measured in cups where the excess can be scraped off the top with a knife.
- Wet ingredients should be measured in a graduated cup so the liquid level can be checked with the eye.

About the Author

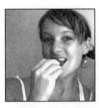 MIELLE CHÉNIER-COWAN ROSE has been a natural foods chef and advocate for natural living for over 15 years, and in the year 2000 she completed the nutritional culinary program at Bauman College in the San Francisco Bay Area. She cut her culinary teeth at Calistoga Natural Cafe, then helped start up a small vegan restaurant in the North Bay and went on to cook at the Macrobiotic Café in Oakland for 3 years. In 2004 she joined Café Gratitude in San Francisco, where she learned more about raw foods and grateful living, and about restaurant management. She self-published the first version of *Vegan*ish in 2011, under the title *Piece of My Heart: A Collection of Vegan Recipes & Cooking Techniques*, while simultaneously healing her young daughter's tooth decay with nutrient-dense animal-based foods. Mielle has seen that food heals—body, mind and spirit—and she strives to integrate the sentiments of the animal rights movement with the realization that some animal-based foods are actually an important element of her family's diet. Readers of her culinary writing can almost taste the uncommon reverence she has for her ingredients, for cooking, and for every being on the planet.

Mielle lives with her daughter in the Sierra foothills of Northern California, where she's delighted to have finally left the noisy chaos of her beloved city life for the quieter chaos of the country. Surrounded and inspired by conscious and talented farmers and foodies, she caters retreats, teaches classes, consults about food and nutrition, coordinates cooking classes at the local co-op community cooking school, and keeps her kitchen at home teeming with interesting projects. Her meals were once compared to the excitement of an amusement park ride, and she works hard to live up to the compliment!